D1282693

Psychobattery

A Chronicle of Psychotherapeutic Abuse

I will use treatment to help the sick according to my ability and judgment, but I will never use it to injure or wrong them.

—Hippocrates

PSYCHOBATTERY

A Chronicle of Psychotherapeutic Abuse

***by* Therese Spitzer**

With medical discussion by
Ralph Spitzer, PhD, MD

Foreword by Joseph Needham

Humana Press. Inc. • Clifton, New Jersey

Dedication

To those humane and scientific doctors and nurses who believe that sound medical treatment and compassionate care are the sine qua non of treating the mentally ill

Library of Congress Cataloging in Publication Data

Main entry under title

Spitzer, Therese.
Psychobattery, a chronicle of psychotherapeutic abuse.

Includes bibliographical references.
1. Mental illness—Physiological aspects—Case studies. 2. Psychotherapy—Complications and sequelae—Case studies. 3. Diagnostic errors—Case studies. I. Spitzer, Ralph. II. Title. [DNLM: 1. Psychotherapy—Case studies. WM420.3 S769p]
RC455.4.B5S64 616.89 79-92083
ISBN 0-89603-014-8

Crescent Manor
P. O. Box 2148
Clifton, NJ 07015

Printed in the United States of America

Table of Contents

Foreword

It is an honour for me to be asked to contribute a foreword to the book of my friends Thérèse and Ralph Spitzer. I got to know them during an assignment as Visiting Professor at the University of British Columbia at Vancouver, and I have shared to the full the distress that comes to all those who have to watch people that they love affected by mental illness in one form or another.

I have been an orientalist for only half my life; for the first half I was a biochemist, embryologist, and experimental morphologist. "When I, a young man, was called to the bar" (as Gilbert & Sullivan have it), in other words, when in the early twenties I was starting life as a research biochemist, I was greatly attracted to the biochemistry of mental disease. I followed the lectures for the Diploma in Psychological Medicine, and worked at the Fulbourn Mental Hospital near Cambridge on the creatinine metabolism in catatonic patients suffering from what we used to call in those days *dementia praecox.* I published one paper (with T. J. McCarthy), but my hopes soon faded, and when I read an excellent review on the subject which covered much literature, and ended by saying that biochemists had grown tired of "fishing in distilled water for the causes of mental disease," I realised that I had better find something more worthwhile. Eggs and embryos were the answer, and very worthwhile they were.

But the decades passed, knowledge increased, and the time came once again when I felt that any young man would be very well advised to go in for neurological and psychological biochemistry. Contemporaries of my own, like Derek Richter and J. H. Quastel, had made pioneer discoveries, and vast new fields were opened up. I followed from a distance the new developments in neuro-anatomy and -physiology, the plotting of previously unimagined neuron connections, often by such delicate methods as fluorescence, and the revelation of pain and pleasure centers in the midbrain, or clumps of neurons concerned with analgesia or hyperalgesia. Gating theories threw light on the perception of pain and its inhibition, and the peripheral connections of the cerebral cortex were mapped out.

Even more revolutionary were the advances in neurochemistry. Many enzymes characteristic of the brain and neural axis were discovered, and, equally important, many of those small molecules that we now call neurotransmitters—serotonin, γ-aminobutyric acid, dopamine, and the like. When I was a medical student, and used to make models of the spinal cord in plasticine, we thought entirely in terms of wire and cable connections, a Post Office telecommunications view, but not we know that the whole nervous system is a mass of minute chemical factories, with the dendrons producing puffs of many different substances acting on the next neuron across the synapse down the line. Otto von Loewy was the father and mother of all this, with his discovery of the effects of acetylcholine on the heart muscle; and now for decades the distinction between cholinergic and adrenergic nerve endings has been a commonplace. Only in the last few years, however, has come the exciting discovery of the endogenously produced opioid peptides, the enkephalins and endorphins, with all their functions, not only in control of pain but probably in many other forms of control and drive also. Yet another chapter has been the unfolding of knowledge about the psychotropic drugs, the hallucinogens, the mood changers (tricyclic and other antidepressants), the tranquilisers, the narcotics and quasi-narcotics—a whole laboratory shelf of powerful agents ranging from the violently dangerous to the enormously beneficient. And some there are too, such as the lithium salts, so valuable in the manic–depressive states, for which as yet no clear theory of action exists, unlike those others which act quite simply as monoamine oxidase inhibitors and so conserve the needed neurotransmitter molecules. And all this is to say nothing of the clearly visualised but yet little known effects on the brain, and hence the mind, of the many hormones of the body, including the newly discovered but powerful prostaglandins.

In parallel with all this there developed the psychological approach, also since the twenties. I always believe that I was fortunate in being a student when A. G. Tansley was expounding the ideas of Sigmund Freud to English readers. The *New Introductory Lectures* I devoured on the long transatlantic sea-voyages of those days. At the B.A.'s table at Caius we talked exclusively of Oedipus complexes, anxiety neuroses, penis envy, and Jungian archetypes, and I believe that this familiarisation was profoundly beneficial to me; otherwise I could have been very alarmed by psychological phenomena that I experienced as I grew older. The *Psycho-Pathology of Everyday Life* was assuredly a great help for many people. I believe that Freud, Adler, and Jung were men of the deepest insight, as revolutionary and liberating in their way as Darwin, Marx, and Huxley had been before them, and I believe too that the cathartic method has been in some cases veritably therapeutic. Subsequent generations, however, developed methods of much more dubious value, greatly in the public eye, and also in psychiatric practice, at the present day. I refer to that sociological psychiatry which sees everything in personal and familial terms, or the group therapies and encounter groups of so many kinds. We may certainly grant that society is far from ideal anywhere, indeed itself deeply sick, especially in the Western world and parts of the Third, but it is not something that the individual citizen, however mentally ill he or she may be, can totally contract out of.

Looking back, I do not think that the purely psychological line of development has anything like the achievements in assured knowledge to its credit which the neurophysiological and neurochemical has, elementary though our understanding is, and for long to come will be. And yet there is a certain dogmatism that insists the troubles of the mind can only be dispelled mentally. This is a denial of the psychophysical interrelation, the organic character of human beings. I suspect also that this prejudice has its roots in a Christianity too much infected by Manichaeism and Gnosticism. "People think of the soul" wrote Middleton Murry, "as if it was a superior little gentleman living on the top floor of a disreputable block of apartments." The *philosophia perennis* of China, always unwilling to separate spirit from matter, never fell into this damaging trap.

What the mind really is, I do not pretend to know. I accept, however, as the only reasonable working hypothesis that all mental events are accompanied by concomitant physicochemical events, even though it will probably take mankind centuries yet to achieve an approximate comprehension of this. At the same time it seems to me that the disturbances inducing mental illness may arise either from the socio-mental level or from the physicochemical level. After all, the same could be said of corporeal illness, for gastric or duodenal ulcer may well follow excessive societal strain, though that could probably not put the interstitial cells of the pancreas out of action. Psychosomatic medicine has certainly come to stay in the West, though the medical systems of Asia have always recognised it. As William Blake wrote nearly two centuries ago:

> Man has no Body distinct from his Soul; for that called Body is a portion of Soul discerned by the five Senses, the chief inlets of Soul in this age.

The idea of the psychophysical organism was never better expressed. And if mental illness may originate either from "above" or from "below," as it were, I am prepared to believe that it may be cured either from above or from below, either by judicious psychoanalytic procedures or by neuropharmacology. Some sort of place must also obviously be left for the phenomena of "faith-healing," difficult though they are to document or to reproduce.

The ocean of troubles described in this book of the Spitzers arises largely from the crass stupidity and gross dogmatism of those who insist that one explanation, one therapy alone, is right. And it must be admitted that most of these doctrinal bigots are on the pharmacophobic side, not the pharmacophilic; in other words they believe they can handle the mind while despising the atoms and molecules with which it is indissolubly associated. As Chêng Ming-Tao said in the 11th century:

> Those who strive to understand the high without studying the low: how can their understanding of the high be right?

It has been my own fate to see individuals whom I loved dominated by the evil power of mental illness. Dora (as I shall name her) I knew first as a student at Girton. Then eventually she married a young man in a government ministry and at first seemed very happy. Some years later I remember sitting with her on a bench in the Green Park in London and sensing that something was profoundly wrong—only a few months later she killed both her children and had to be certified insane. No on was more surprised than her psychiatrist, who had supposed she was suffering from mild neurotic symptoms. Often have I wondered whether neuropharmacology could not have prevented that tragedy. Many years later there was Sophie, a learned and even eminent French scholar, who fell into a deep depression with complete loss of libido and suicidal ruminations. Like so many humanists, and indeed ordinary people today, she was a true pharmacophobe, and would rather have the headache than the aspirin; indeed they often can be heard to say "I never take medicines—just natural things like marijuana." Fortunately, here the ending was a happy one, for new high responsibilities and the disappearance of certain embarrassing relationships brought about a complete return to health. And other situations have been resolved happily too; dear Susan, for example, kept on an even keel with antidepressants for years; and from my experience with students as the head of a Cambridge College, I know the power of these medicines.

Thus I sincerely hope that the book of the Spitzers will make people realise that fashionable psychology and psychiatry are not alone the answer. Always the underlying physicochemical mechanisms should be looked for. Quite apart from the subtle malfunctions of neurochemistry, all sorts of things can cause mental abnormality—spirochetes, trypanosomes, porphyrin metabolism, pancreatic, pulmonary and cerebral tumours, multiple sclerosis, hypo- and hyperthyroidism, and many more. My own brother-in-law will bear witness of this; he once contracted a nasty dermatological complaint, for which the general opinion was he would have to be deeply psychoanalysed, until someone thought of asking him whether he cultivated primulas. He did, he stopped, the allergy ceased, and everything cleared up like magic. This was a parallel to the much more dreadful example of familial periodic paralysis, which is now known to depend on faulty ionic balances. But how much suffering has been caused, one wonders, by the blithe assumption of the psychologists that their patients' minds are disembodied. And furthermore how much unnecessary suffering has been caused to perfectly innocent parents and relatives of patients when the mental disease of the subject has been confidently attributed to failure on their part.

I would not wish to seem to be against all psychoanalysis or introspective psychology, or even to deny all value to the weirder forms of psychological shock-therapy current today; but one absolute requisite is that the medical therapeutic urge should be there, not just a dallying with strange psychological phenomena. And this means compassion, the Hippocratic urge. I was much amused many years ago by a slogan in the *New Yorker* "Leave your mind alone!" There is still much to be said for it. At all events, I think that the Spitzers are absolutely right in putting first things first, and where the mind is concerned, the body and its chemistry has a certain primacy. What was it John Donne wrote?

> To our bodies turne wee then, that so
> Weake men on love reveal'd may looke;
> Love's mysteries in soules doe growe
> But yet the body is his booke.

June, 1980

Joseph Needham, FRS, FBA
Cambridge University

Medical Author's Note to the Reader

Several readers of our manuscript have asked me why the chapter on The Biology of Mental Illness was placed fifth instead of first.

As a teacher of medical students, who are highly motivated to understand why things work, I have found that my teaching is much more successful when it is introduced empirically by first presenting a patient who suffers the condition to be discussed. After the students have examined and spoken to the patient, they are much more receptive to information about the causes and to a scientific explanation of the underlying pathology. Observation of the real patient also prepares their minds to retain the scientific information in a way that appears quite impossible when only abstract concepts and descriptions are presented first.

It is for this reason that we offer several detailed case histories before giving the scientific discussion. In the initial four chapters, several kinds of mental disease whose disabling symptoms mental health professionals are trying to control are thoroughly illustrated; some of the widely used medications are also introduced, along with accounts of their benefits and harmful side effects. It is my belief that the chapter on the Biology of Mental Illness will be much more meaningful after this introduction.

However, different people learn differently. Some people, of a deductive turn of mind, prefer to have as much theoretical information as possible before addressing concrete examples. In this way they feel better able to correlate the observable manifestations with the scientific background, and thus more completely understand the clinical condition.

To those readers who prefer the second method of developing understanding, I would suggest reading Chapter 5 first. It stands reasonably well on its own, and checking an occasional cross-reference ought redress any deficiencies.

Acknowledgments

My thanks go, first, to Theresa Galloway, whose encouragement led to the conversion of what was simply a file of cases into the present narrative. Then, to those courageous parents, spouses, and patients who wanted the stories of their sufferings told that others might be spared. The prowess of my research assistant, Sue Yates, is shown by her finding, in ten minutes, a New Yorker article of which I knew neither the title, the author nor the year of publication. Anna Leith, Director of the Woodward Biomedical Library, was most helpful. My interest in the whole field was greatly stimulated by my two great Boston teachers: Dr. Abigail Adams Eliot, psychologist, and Dr. Robert Hyde, psychiatrist. I have benefited greatly from conversations with Professor James Taylor, whose legal knowledge is exceeded only by his compassion. Finally, the book would not have been possible without the help of my editor and publisher, Thomas Lanigan, who gently helped me to convert a collection of case histories into a book.

1

What *Psychobattery* is About

September 5, 19—

Dear Sandy,

Sorry I haven't written for so long, but I've been going through really hard times. I hesitate to write even now, because this letter will probably depress you, but here goes.

In August, I started getting really depressed. Sue had left for Philadelphia and I had been spending most of my time with her before she left. Well, I spent a month and a half lying around in my bedroom, and just coming down for meals. I was really sad and I thought about suicide most of the time.

Then in September my parents suggested that I go to the Teaching Hospital Day Care Program, so I went. This consisted of very heavy encounter sessions—3 or 4 hours a day—and then Occupational Therapy and sports the rest of the time. The encounter groups were very painful, but I supposed that the program would do me some good and I was led to understand that I could not remain in it without participation in groups.

Anyway, the whole thing exploded on Monday (5 days ago). We had a particularly hellish encounter group where I was told I was like a little child and that I was too friendly. It brought home to me that I was a drag on my family and that my mother's rapidly greying hair was my fault. It felt like a bad acid trip, with dripping faces, distortions, and colors. I went home, cried for two hours, and took all the pills I had, since I just couldn't go on any longer.

Well, they found out, rushed to the drugstore to get an emetic, which I took and vomited up the capsules, and so here I am.

I'm really happy about you and Steve—I love both of you and think you go really well together.

Well that's all.

Love,
Frank

This verbatim letter (except for changes of names, dates, and places) outlines the difficult, widespread, and often literally life and death problem we shall deal with throughout this book. A sensitive young man has been ill for about four years and puts himself in professional hands when he needs help with a serious and life-threatening depression. He asks for bread and receives a stone—in the form of aggressive group therapy leading to a serious suicide attempt.

Encounter therapy is one of many current "group therapies" that attempt to cure by encouraging patients to relive their pasts and re-experience all the angers and hostilities they may ever have felt in their family environments. In some variants the hostility is expressed by striking people with styrofoam bats or objects with more solid weapons. "When I 'came to'" said Joan Rayburn, a retired school teacher, who was directed by her therapist to express anger against her dead father by beating a pillow, "my hands were bloody from the force with which I had wielded the hammer."

Even with people who are only mildly disturbed (and who therefore do not fall into the category of those suffering from mental illness, as we have defined it below), it is now being found that therapies of this type have a high incidence of deleterious effects, expressed in various papers as a 10–20% casualty rate. This high incidence of harm should be widely known so that people who choose to pursue this form of treatment may be aware of the dangerous voyage they are embarking on.

The concern in *Psychobattery* is not, however, with people who are lonely, sad, dissatisfied, or maladjusted, although I sympathize with them and appreciate their problems. I am agonized by the plight of the truly mentally ill; those people who at some time in their lives have experienced a change that makes it impossible for them to function in society. The change may be one that causes any of a range of problems, from sleeplessness, loss of appetite and self-esteem, and the feeling of being weighted down as by an enormous stone, to preoccupation with suicide as the only way out. At the other extreme from these depressed patients are the manic—euphoric, buoyant, moving and talking too fast to be comprehended, full of grandiose schemes that change daily or hourly, not eating because of a lack of time rather than of appetite. They may die of malnutrition, sleep deprivation, exposure to the elements, or as the result of a particularly bad misjudgment in some activity normally safe. Another type of patient, the schizophrenic, undergoes an even more serious change in personality, beginning perhaps with misperceptions and hallucinations, and ending in withdrawal from reality and society. In between, schizophrenics lose their jobs, friends, enjoyment of life, and possibly, with the help of some misguided "therapists," also their families, which under other circumstances might have provided the only support available.

These medically ill people can often be helped by medical treatment. There are medications that are more or less specific for each of the symptoms described above. Alternating manic–depressive illness can be virtually abolished. In the less tractable schizophrenias, ameliorative medication may make it possible for the patient to take an interest in life, to live outside the hospital, to establish some relationships and, in a few cases, to go back to, or to begin, work.

The cruel and fundamental error constantly illustrated in the case histories we present here is the assumption that all these disastrous illnesses are caused primarily by some flaw in parental personality or family dynamics, and that their proper treatment lies in dwelling on these familial unpleasantnesses, incidents that occur in every family, but are totally disregarded when no one becomes ill. The result is guilt, unhappiness, alienation, suffering, and—even worse—neglect of medical treatment that might be of real benefit.

We are fortunately in the midst of a great debate on this problem—a debate whose venue ranges from the pages of scholarly papers such as *Psychiatry and Psychotherapy: Is a Divorce Imminent*?,[1] to the Monday morning seminars of university psychiatry departments, to the pages of *Time* magazine and even of the *TV Guide*. More and more it is being stated by professors of psychiatry, medical writers in the lay press, psychologists, and others that these illnesses are biological and subject to biological treatment. That the psychological "therapies," far from being innocuous, are often positively unhelpful, carrying high casualty rates, even for *normal volunteers*. It is my concern that such potentially harmful, and even lethal, treatments should not be applied to seriously ill mental patients, who already have problems enough and who, even if they have volunteered for hospital admission rather than being committed, really have no choice about accepting whatever therapy may be proferred. Patients in mental hospitals, in contrast to those in any other type of hospital, have no choice of physician, and they are frequently threatened with eviction from the hospital or with involuntary legal committal if they do not accept suggested treatment. Of course, no one accepts responsibility (or may even be aware) when the forcibly voluntary treatment results in failure, or indeed, suicide (see Chapter 10).

The case histories and discussion in the remainder of the book will illustrate these points.

The reader might like to know how I became interested in this problem.

Years ago, when I interned in clinical psychology at a famous New England center for emotionally disturbed children, I made clinical contact with my first autistic child. From the age of six months, the child had exhibited ever-increasing abnormalities. He rocked in his crib and banged his head. Although he never spoke, he would scream meaninglessly for hours on end. Unable to sit up or crawl, he suddenly started walking at age two. He never learned to play with toys or with other children, nor did he show that he recognized their existence.

The desperate parents traveled half way across the United States to get help for their child. They were informed, gently, that the cause of their child's catastrophic illness lay in the mother's unconscious cold rejection of him. I can still recall her bewilderment as she tried to comprehend what she had done to her child. A short time after they left the Center, she killed herself.

According to the theory advanced by the Center's psychotherapeutic personnel, this mother should have been characterized by obsessive personality and emotional frigidity. My observation of her simply did not fit this description. She seemed a perfectly normal mother, distraught with suffering. She wept during an interview and, under the ministration of the psychoanalytic theorists, began to doubt whether her love and concern were "real."

Although this one example was not sufficient to destroy my established faith in a theory that was taught with all the dogmatism of revealed religion, I was badly shaken by its obvious inhumanity in application and by its destructive consequence to this unfortunate mother. Neither, at the time, did I realize that there was no scientific basis for the coarse and painful experimentation with families that grew out of such hypotheses, no adequate "methods for clinical assessment." And yet serious papers and books, which I read avidly, were being written on maternal deprivation as the cause of autism and childhood schizophrenia. In short, "These theories and practices produced guilt-consumed parents of psychotic children."[2]

Ten years later, the daughter of a dear friend developed ulcerative colitis. As though her illness were not tragic enough, the family was subjected to long years of psychiatric inquisition to find the source of the family conflict that had caused the child's colonic mucosa to shred away in bleeding strips, ultimately leading to her death from cancer. Since I knew the family intimately and knew there was no serious conflict, either hidden or open, my doubts about such types of psychotherapy began to extend to the theories on which they were based.

In later years, when I led discussion groups for mothers, under the auspices of Family Services or various school boards, or when I taught university courses in "The Changing Family," I became aware of the frequency with which my students had suffered similar incidents. Gradually it dawned upon me that this sort of abuse was very common, and there was little if any, social or medical protection from it. And I began then to realize that mental patients and their families were the most frequent victims of this kind of destructive treatment. With this discouraging realization as my strong motive, I then began recording interviews with these doubly-victimized families and found that the very act of chronicling their encounters with the psychotherapeutic community clarified my own views of the mischievous processes at work, and in time led to the writing of this book.

When my interest became known, many people volunteered for interviews and often sent friends or relatives who had been victimized. Although they wanted their histories used to prevent similar trauma to others, most of them were not eager to be identified since they feared they might be made to suffer more on their next encounter with a psychiatric "team," or therapist, or on admission to a mental hospital. Therefore, in order to protect them, changes have been made in the names and personal data of the patients and families in this book. The doctors and other agents of these misguided therapies who provided treatment have been thoroughly amalgamated, and are here designated by pseudonyms, thus protecting the guilty as well as the innocent. Every effort has been made to preserve the privacy of all concerned, in recognition of both the legal and the moral imperatives involved.

The bulk of the book consists of excerpts from these interviews. In addition to the description of the unsympathetic, harmful, and often brutal treatment meted out to these patients and their families—most of which I am convinced is based on unproved and unprovable hypotheses—there is also discussion of other theories of mental illness and examples of how, in some cases, their application leads to more satisfactory outcomes.

Each chapter uses a primary patient case history to illustrate certain basic points. Subsidiary issues may be brought in by vignettes from other case histories. Each chronicle is then followed by or interwoven with a discussion of the theories on which the many varieties of mistreatment are based and, whenever possible, a more humane and possibly satisfactory management of the disease is suggested.

The medical portions of this book have been checked or written by my husband, Dr. Ralph Spitzer, a chemical pathologist and university professor of pathology of long standing, who has made a special study of the biology of mental illness as a result of our mutual interest in this subject.

It is our hope that the material in this book will help protect the thousands of sufferers from mental illness and their families from the well-meaning but inept attempts of fad-ridden therapists, and will lead to a more humane and effective therapy, administered by a medical profession that has properly returned to its medical base.

2

Savage Encounter

> No patient should be worse for
> having seen a doctor.
> —Willie Evans

Greta Thomas was the third and last child in her family. She was extremely pretty, and very popular, and in her early teens she never lacked dates. The change in her personality began sometime in her fifteenth year, when she became depressed and withdrawn.

> I dreamt about suicide. I felt so worthless and useless—then I started drinking because it made me feel good and I liked it.

When she was seventeen, her father died and her family life was thereafter disrupted. The older siblings married, leaving Greta and her mother at home together. Then at nineteen, Greta married, but the marriage lasted scarcely beyond the honeymoon. She was drinking very heavily by this time in an attempt to escape from her terrible depressions and suicidal dreams. Since she was an extremely artistic person, she was at that time still able to eke out a living between bouts with the bottle and with depression. During the next few years, however, she made several suicide bids that fortunately were thwarted by family and friends. At twenty-eight she remarried, but the new relationship was rather a rocky one because of her drinking and her frequently depressed state of mind. A year later, Greta made another suicide attempt that landed her in the university teaching hospital.

Much of my poignant interview with her follows:

Question: Let's begin with some of your observations about the teaching hospital and your experiences there.
Greta: Well, they seem to do a great deal of experimenting there. Twice I was interviewed, once by a nurse and once by a doctor, while other people watched through a one-way mirror just to be able to grade the interviewer's technique. One time I was interviewed by my doctor. Dr. Ayrs, who is the head there, and four or five medical students were watching through the one-way mirror. After the interview was finished, the doctor who had interviewed me was waiting in the hall. Dr. Ayrs asked if I would like to come in with them to listen to the interview, and I said, "All right." So I went in and the medical students then each gave their opinion of the interviewing technique, as did Dr. Ayrs, who then turned to me and asked the medical students to give their own opinions of me—of what I would be like as a wife! I said, "Why a wife?" And he said, "Oh well—you know—" and evaded the question. So I sat there and listened to each one of them give their opinions of me—you know, what they would think of me as a wife, and I couldn't believe what was going on because, after all, why *do* people get married? But anyway there was one doctor, one intern, who refused to comment, and I thought he was very brave because Dr. Ayrs was there like a hawk, wanting them all to give their opinions.
Question: Did Dr. Ayrs give his opinion of you as a wife?
Greta: Yes. He didn't think I'd be too hot. I can't remember everything he said, except that it was all derogatory. And he did say he thought I was the kind of person who, if you brought me a dozen long-stemmed roses, would complain that they weren't short-stemmed. That seemed pretty ridiculous to me, and humiliating.

It was while I was still a patient there that I first heard about Therapy House. It was Dr. Ayrs who recommended that I apply there, and when I was about to be discharged from the Teaching Hospital, I did. First I went to the therapist working there, who asked me various questions, and then said that I would have to be voted in by the patients at Therapy House at that time. I agreed to appear before them since I felt that Therapy House might be able to help me, and I went there to be interviewed by the group. The meeting was held in the theatre and the patients sat in a semicircle around the new applicants who had come to be either accepted or rejected by the house. They took us one at a time and they asked us questions such as: "Are you on medication?" I said, "Yes, I am," and they told me that if I went into Therapy House I would be off all medication. They told me that I would have to be strongly committed to the group five days a week for the six full weeks that I'd go to Therapy House, and for the tapering off period, too.

Question: Would you go back for a moment, Greta? What was meant by being "strongly committed to the group"?

Greta: Well, I understood it to be not going against group rules, such as not being late, not taking medication, not drinking, not fraternizing outside with group members, and if I broke a commitment to make up for it, and other such things. But it seemed to go a lot deeper than that. If you objected to some of the rules, for example, to having your family members at family night, that was counted as being against the group, and you were therefore said not to be committed to the group, and the members gave you static. And if you objected to any of their so-called therapy—several times I thought it was rather cruel what they were doing to some of the people there....

Question (after waiting for Greta to go on): Can you give an example of this cruelty?

Greta: I remember maybe three or so. There was one girl there whose eyes were crossed, and who was very self-conscious over that. The group felt that she was unable to stand up for herself, that she wasn't assertive enough, and that one of the reasons she wasn't assertive was that when she was a child, the other children in school had teased her about her eyes, as apparently everybody else in her life has done since! So the group took on roles, and began taunting her, and pushing and shoving her, and hitting her with the bopper.

Question: The bopper?

Greta: It was sort of club with a handle to grasp—it was a foam-padded bat was what it was—and it was used for "therapeutic" purposes to hit people, forcing them to react. That's what they were doing to her, and finally she got angry. They felt she had made progress because the girl had gotten angry at the teasing about her eyes. They said that in her anger she was expressing assertiveness, and therefore was making progress. Of course, then she started crying, and she couldn't stop until she was exhausted and had curled up on a mat by herself.

Another time they had a girl down on the floor questioning her about her sex life, and things like that, because her father had molested her when she was a child. They were trying to get her to express her anger against her father and I felt they were quite rough with her. They kept yelling at her to open up, you know. And they said, "Tell us how he fucked you!"

One other time—it was on a Friday—excuse me, I can't remember all the instances—but there was one girl who was resisting the group's efforts to get her angry and react. She kept retreating and retreating, and was walking away from everybody with the boppers. Finally we all took turns at this bopping business, and the people got tired and I was bopping her and suddenly the idea of hitting people to help them sounded ridiculous. Anyway I was bopping her, and suddenly *I* was angry. Something snapped inside me—here I was hitting this girl! I wasn't even thinking of her as a person any more. It affected me very strongly. I remember it happened just before Therapy House was over—it was on a Friday, and I was going away for the weekend. We went, and I couldn't function for practically the whole weekend. I was just so depressed—really depressed—because I'd been hitting that girl.

Question: Was all the "therapy" initiated by the group?
Greta: Oh no. I remember I was sitting in my family group one day and Dr. Breugel, the head of Therapy House sat down with my family. He made a practice of spreading his time around among all of the families. This time he had gotten us all speaking gibberish, which is like speaking in tongues, I guess, and there was a person who was very shy and who withdrew from speaking in gibberish. He said he felt too foolish; he just couldn't do it. And I remember I found it very difficult to do too, and although I did it, I felt like a complete fool. And he was refusing to go along with the group. So the doctor maneuvered him into standing up on a chair, and we all sat around on the floor looking up at him and forced him, because of our zeroing him out, to speak gibberish. And Dr. Breugel said to him, "You really think you are superior, don't you!" Finally the man of course spoke in gibberish. I imagine it was quite painful for him to do that. He couldn't look at us after Dr. Breugel had put him down; he just mumbled and really seemed dazed all the rest of the day.

I am often haunted by what might have happened to him—he was such a quiet, undemonstrative person. I know that one of our group, a nurse, committed suicide a year later.
Question: What other "therapy" methods were used?
Greta: Breaking people down seemed to be the most important approach. Usually it started with verbal assault, and then the boppers would be brought out and people would be hit. Or sometimes it would happen after they read their autobiographies, into which we had usually put our whole souls because we were supposed to be committed to the group and to reveal *all.* Then we would be led to mats and made to lie down. And the group would hold the person down and ask questions that they knew from earlier sessions would be quite painful. People would resist. Very personal questions; and the group encouraged a person to resist. They might scream at the person on the mat, get angry, or say something like: What

do you really think of your father? What do you really think of your mother? And the person would break down. When it happened to me, it was almost like losing consciousness. You're not even aware after a while that the people around you are screaming at you, and often you find yourself crying. I found the whole thing quite shocking.

I remember one time when a girl was "working on the mat," that's when you just lie down on a mat and kick and scream and yell and sort of make primal screams. This girl was crying out for her father, who had died when she was a young girl. Everyone thought she was making progress because she was at last exorcising all her anger and frustration at her father for dying when she had been so young. I questioned that. I wondered about the value of it—but you grow used to accepting psychiatric methods without question after a while—it's a species of brainwashing, I guess . . . Of course if you cried when you were working on the mat, you were a grand success—then there were enormous displays of contrived emotion and hugging afterwards . . .

Question: Did Dr. Breugel supervise this?

Greta: He'd encourage it. In fact whenever he was in the theatre with all of us as a group, it was as if a signal for a mass breakdown had been given because that was his bag, was what he wanted. I imagine he really believed that it was beneficial. One day, he told us that he was thinking of constructing a capsule room, soundproof, where someone would be away from any stimulus except for a tape recorder that would play a word or phrase repeatedly. He was wondering whether this would be therapeutically beneficial. "We are human engineers," he often said.

We did a great deal of role-playing too. At various times, different members of the group were chosen to play the mother or the father or whatever. But sometimes the characters weren't madly in love with one another, to say the least. If I took a role in which I had a problem with my dead father (which at the time they convinced me that I did have), and if *in that role* I hated my father, and if there was someone in the group I didn't like, then he would usually play my father. He would act out this role with redoubled emotion, and I found that very disturbing. I remember that once, when I was contemplating separating from my husband, a fellow that I didn't like played my husband, and we screamed at each other back and forth, and he used the bopper and was extremely abusive. I wound up hating my husband even more than I had before playing this little psychodrama.

Question: Did the patients' families ever visit Therapy House?

Greta: Oh, yes. Once a week we had family night and the patient group would stay past four-thirty waiting for the family members to arrive. We all gathered in the theatre and the visiting family member would sit on the stage with his member of the group while the rest of the group sat in a circle around the stage and asked the family visitor any question at all—it didn't matter how personal.

Question: Greta, when you refer to "family member" you mean someone who was not under psychiatric treatment, someone who was just a family member of the patient. Is that correct?

Greta: Yes, a relative of the member of the group, or a friend that someone had brought to family night. The group would ask them all sorts of questions—any questions at all, nothing was out of bounds—in the guise of helping the member of the group. There was role-playing in that process, too. For instance, if the mother of one member of the group had come and was sitting on the stage, any member of the group could run up and stand behind the mother, speaking for her, and saying anything he or she wished. Or they might stand behind the group member as well, speaking on the member's behalf. It was often rather humiliating for those family members who hadn't realized what they were getting into. For instance, that girl whose father had died when she was young had a problem with her mother. At least, the group thought that she did. When the mother came to family night, she got quite a going over. Everyone role-played and spoke for her, telling her that she was competing sexually with her daughter, or that she had never accepted the fact that her daughter had grown up. I wonder how she found the courage to come back again!

Question: Did your own mother come to family night?

Greta: No, she didn't need any more pain. Of course, the group felt that I wasn't living up to my commitment when I didn't produce her, and they really put me down for that.

Question: What was the outcome of your experiences at Therapy House?

Greta: Well, before I first transferred there from the hospital, they insisted on a commitment not to take any medication. But I'd been on medication in the hospital for some time before that. Therapy House had the hospital records, and should have known that I had been in there as a patient for drinking, that I'd decided to stop drinking, and joined AA, and gone on medication. But when I went to Therapy House, they made me stop medication altogether. Stopping drinking isn't easy; neither is stopping medication, especially when I needed it and especially when I was going through the traumatic experience of Therapy House itself. I was supposed to attend some tapering off sessions after finishing full-time at Therapy House, but I couldn't because by that time I was just starting the worst breakdown in my experience. It lasted severely for six months, and it's still affecting me in the sense that I'm much more nervous than I was before. I have since been warned that if I don't stay on medication I'll be in hospital for the rest of my life. So I feel that Therapy House is directly responsible for my breakdown.

Question: Have you worked since your breakdown?

Greta: When I finally left the hospital after the breakdown, I didn't work for some time because I simply couldn't. I finally found a job in January, at the local Art

> Gallery, and after working there for a while, I did some work as an illustrator. I'm now taking a design course and trying never to have another breakdown. I have to stay on my medication. I'd *never* go into a place like Therapy House again and am hoping I'll stay out of hospital.

Greta was put on Mellaril (an antipsychotic) during her hospitalization at the time of her last breakdown. Since then her depression has been managed successfully with lithium and Mellaril.

For Greta, therapy was a destructive process, and only psychoactive drugs allowed her to live a semblance of a normal life. But drugs of course are not always the best alternative, and where they do prove helpful they must be carefully monitored. Thus, a great deal of concern has been expressed—by some psychiatrists as well as some mental patients—about the dangers of long term use of phenothiazines (Mellaril is a phenothiazine). The most serious long-term effect is *tardive dyskinesia,* a nervous defect in which the patient develops symptoms similar to Parkinson's Disease; that is, tremors, rigidity, posturing, etc. Tardive dyskinesia is indeed a serious disease. And it is, at the moment, incurable. However, the incidence is dose related, and at the small dosage being taken by Greta, her chance of developing the disease is probably less than 1%. Patients taking very large doses for many years have a higher probability, as do patients over fifty.

The problem of side effects is not unique to psychopharmacology. Virtually any medication used in chronic illness has possibly deleterious side effects. The probability of such side effects must be taken into consideration along with the benefits, and it is up to the patient to make an informed decision, which is really a choice of the lesser of two evils. Greta is fully informed about her choice and feels that she would much rather take what is, for her, a small risk of developing dyskinesia than accept the virtual certainty of becoming a permanent hospital patient.

Greta used the term "brainwashing" when she was discussing the mental patient's sensitivity to the suggestions of the therapist, but this receptiveness is naturally derived from the patient's earlier experiences. It is quite normal in all societies for patients to trust the judgment of the medical personnel who are treating their physical disabilities. They recognize that the aim of such treatment is the restoration of the whole person to health, and expect that this will be the aim of all treatments undertaken or prescribed by a physician. It is highly to be regretted, therefore, that this very trust was precisely what prevented the patients at Therapy House from recognizing that their treatment regime could produce the opposite effect, a fragmentation and disintegration of the personality.

Greta is not the only patient of Therapy House who suffered from her experiences. Dorothy Herman discussed her experiences there, but only with some reluctance:

> I suffered such personality collapse after Therapy House that I haven't been able to work since.
>
> The processes of breaking down, all that screaming and thrashing—people shouting, "Daddy, daddy!"—was simply terrifying! I'd gone into Therapy House because I was depressed. I needed to gain control over my emotions, to obtain help in sorting out the hang-ups in my marriage. But I found that this business of being open and writing a daily diary led only to harassment. The group members questioned me about things that I found too personal to discuss, and they zeroed in on sensitive matters like sex with such venom that sometimes I *did* break down and scream just like they wanted. They tried to make me direct my anger against my mother and my husband—and I did. In the end, my marriage did break up—Therapy House made sure of that.
>
> I just can't stop being haunted by the fact that I had my mother travel all the way from the east for family night just to be crucified! For weeks after Therapy House I

> couldn't talk to anyone. I shook all the time, and I started to drink. Before I went to Therapy House, I was no more than a social drinker, but afterwards it didn't take me long to become an alcoholic. I became so fearful of people, I couldn't go back to work. Then, when I'd nearly hit the bottom, a friend took me to Alcoholics Anonymous. That's been a good experience, and maybe in time I'll feel like my old self again.

In a specialty one always imagines to be characterized by sensitivity, empathy, and compassion for the sufferer, it is alarming to see how many incidents in Greta's and Dorothy's stories are based on the humiliation and debasement of the patient. In particular, Greta's story of her own humiliation as the interns discussed her suitability as a wife is extremely poignant. Equally disturbing is the evident suggestibility of the young medical students, who entered all too easily into the demeaning and insensitive spirit of the attending psychiatrist's suggestion. Only one intern had the moral presence of mind to refuse to rate her, saying that her case wasn't sufficiently well elaborated that an opinion could legitimately be formed.

What of the young man who was forced to mount the chair when he wouldn't speak in gibberish, and of the girl who was taunted and "bopped" because her eyes were "crossed"? How could any of those events have helped the patients to regain a state of mental health in which they could once again appropriately control their minds and emotions?

Patients seldom fight to save themselves. Even when Greta had been humiliated, she didn't express her feelings to Dr. Ayrs and the interns. And the young man never hit Dr. Breugel for making him stand on the stool as though he were a child. Nobody had suggested bringing out the boppers when the doctors were instigating the patients' humiliations.

The acquiescence of both of these patients demonstrated their flexibility in the face of authoritarian commands—behavior that would no doubt have been condemned by these same psychiatrists if a parent had used it on a child. It is important for the psychiatrists involved to realize that the patients forgave them—once the initial humiliation and anger had passed—even as these patients had forgiven their parents long ago in similar situations.

How could psychiatrists imagine that such methods help patients to gain genuine control over their lives? Especially such modest and reserved people as most psychotics are? Dr. Philip Zimbardo,[1] an eminent social psychologist at Stanford University, has said that "if you insult and embarrass a shy person who is psychotic, then you make that person shy *and* crazy."

The "voting" process to which the patient must be subjected in order to be admitted to Therapy House is also open to question. Is the power the group feels in the rejection or acceptance of a patient a healthy feeling? Does the patient who is rejected suffer an additional loss of self-esteem and self-worth? Is there follow-up to see how he fared? One patient who said she felt suicidal was attacked by a doctor who screamed, "Get out! You promised you wouldn't commit suicide if you came into the group, now get out!" What happened to her?

Unfortunately, even as this book goes to press, Therapy House still does not conduct followup studies once its patients have left, so that there are no statistics on rehospitalization, suicides, or recovery after treatment.

We should consider one further aspect of encounter therapy. Greta says that something snapped in her when she found herself hitting the other patient repeatedly. She became so angry that she "wasn't thinking of her as a person anymore." Is it possible that evoking uncontrolled emotions that lead to the use of physical force can be an appropriate "treatment" for mental patients? I suggest that this is not only dangerous to mental health, but that it is at best ethically questionable for the medical profession to cause such disorientation and lack of control.

An interesting question about the effect of using violence as a therapeutic modality is raised by a recently printed story.

A psychiatric nurse in a hospital in which boppers were used came home from his day's work and beat his long-time friend and housemate four times over the head with a hammer. The friend, who was sleeping at the time, received cuts and head injuries.

The attacker was tried, convicted, granted a suspended sentence, and ordered on probation for two years. The judge apparently considered the attack as partially excusable because the nurse had been under severe emotional strain caused by the suicide of two of his patients that very day.

There is no way to prove or disprove that this nurse's experience in soliciting violence had influenced his response to the stress of his job. In my opinion, it is a very strange reaction indeed to the sadness generated by the suicide of two patients.

In this era, when many organizations are complaining bitterly about violence in the media, when we are trying very hard to erase the battered child and the battered wife syndromes, it seems extremely odd that disturbed people and mental patients should be encouraged to vent their frustration by violent means, either symbolic or real.

3

Primal Scream

Eric Swanson was recently interviewed in depth. The occasion was not suitable for tape recording, and the following data are taken from the interviewer's notes.

Eric is now thirty-five years old and has suffered from schizophrenia for fourteen years. He came to this country when he was eighteen. Having been raised in a disciplined environment, he prided himself on his self-discipline and his high moral principles. He entered university to study forestry and graduated four years later with first class marks. Since he did not believe is socializing, he had made no friends there and had never dated a girl. All his time had been devoted to his studies.

After graduation, he found a job with a large forest products concern, but soon returned to the university to take postgraduate work, this time in the fine arts. After a few months of study, however, he began to experience constant fatigue and to suffer from blurred vision. He went to the university opthalmologist who examined his eyes and then, in Eric's own words:

> He insulted me publicly in front of a whole waiting room full of people! He said I was a lazy bum and that there was nothing wrong with me. He said, "You're rotten! You just don't want to work!" And he told me to go out and get a job.

He then referred Eric to a psychiatrist. Dr. Lake, the psychiatrist, laid the blame for Eric's problems on his own shoulders because of his inability to have fun. Eric recalled the interview with shame:

> "Have you ever had a woman?" Dr. Lake asked me.
> "NO!" I told him proudly.
> "My God!" he yelled at me. "You're the worst case of sexual repression I've ever met!"
> He went on attacking me mercilessly until I just fell apart. I hadn't pleased him. He absolutely rejected me!

At about this time, Eric began to take some courses in physical education and as usual made excellent marks. He also met and married a young woman. He and his wife moved to a small city where he had accepted a job with the parks board. It was not long, however, before Eric found himself unable to cope with the job. He couldn't get up in the morning, he couldn't leave the house alone, and he became afraid of people. His wife took over his job with the parks board. Eric returned to the city to another psychiatrist, Dr. Bailen for help. Dr. Bailen listened to him for three appointments, then according to Eric:

> She ripped me apart! She yelled at me, "You are chickening out! Did you marry your mommy? Go back and take over that job from your wife!" She told me I was running scared of life and that I just needed a kick in the pants to get going.

Eric returned with the resolve to follow the doctor's orders, but within the year he gave up again, and he and his wife returned to the city to move in with her family. This quickly proved unsatisfactory, so they found their own apartment. Eric's wife now took an office job while he worked in day care centers. Finally, unable to cope with his moods, his wife left him. He tried the hippy scene for a while, but soon became disillusioned with their lifestyle. "No one in that culture commits himself to anyone else," he said. But at twenty-six he was no closer to coping with his disintegrating life than he'd been when he first saw Dr. Lake.

It was at this point that he found his third psychiatrist, Dr. Isaacs, who at least encouraged him to hang in there when he felt like ending it all. But after four long years of individual therapy sessions, both Dr. Isaacs and Eric concluded that no progress had been made. However, the doctor did recommend that Eric should approach Dr. Dennison, who was practicing the group encounter technique. He waited two months for an appointment, but afterwards he felt the experience had been worth the delay.

> Dr. Dennison was the first psychiatrist who didn't blame me! He accepted me, he let me talk. And he was warm. I felt taken care of, I trusted him!

For a full month of private sessions, Dr. Dennison listened to him, then at last prescribed medication that calmed him down. He told him to forget the past—throw it away—because they would only talk about the present, the here-and-now.

Eric started taking amphetamines on his own about this time, and found he had tremendous energy; he read the whole of *Bleak House* in a day. But whenever he stopped taking it, he experienced terrible depression. At the end of six more months of private sessions with Dr. Dennison, Eric was introduced to the doctor's encounter group. It was led by Ms. Nancy Haley, a psychologist who used confrontation techniques.

As a prerequisite to membership in the group, as in the Therapy House, each patient was required to be open and honest. Nancy mocked those who found it difficult to be completely open as "phonies." She told them that they did not want to take their lives seriously. Eric opened himself to the group.

> I remember once that I was lying on the floor and they were all screaming at me. And Nancy yelled, "Get off your mother trip!" She nailed me for crying, and she tortured me whenever I opened up. So I retreated more deeply into my natural privacy; I began to lie and to pretend that I was okay.

For the next eighteen months, Eric remained with the group and he learned to play the "group-game" well. There were two kinds of players: those who condemned others, and those who were condemned. Eric, of course joined the condemning side because he knew he couldn't take the condemnation meted out by the other side.

Many of the "therapies" that are discussed in this book seem to lean on the scapegoat principle. Apparently the therapists have discovered that a good way to develop esprit de corps is to single out some member of the group who is aberrant (by definition, usually). In such groups, the deviants are generally those whose feelings of privacy will not allow them to bare their souls to strangers, who then will develop group solidarity by attacking the exposed ones. This is a widespread technique from which we feel no good has, or can ever, come. From the burning of the witches in the middle ages and to the burning of the Jews in Nazi Germany, the unification of a group by leading it to attack a scapegoat has coincided with deterioration in character and in society, and worse. Many of the patients in these groups have recognized the dangers of the technique and have expressed this recognition. The "therapists," alas, have not.

Each week when he attended the group session, Eric pretended to be doing better and better. He persuaded the group to believe that he had found a job and a place to live, and that he was learning to handle his problems. Nancy would hold him up as an example to the rest of the group. But within, Eric was falling apart.

A day came when he could no longer maintain the deception. Dr. Dennison had announced his intention to come to the group that day after a prolonged absence. It was to be his last visit because he was terminating his work with the group. Although the group did not know it, Dr. Dennison was shifting his interest to Primal Scream therapy. He was abandoning his concern for the here-and-now for the there-and-then.

Eric was desperate. He was irrevocably tied to Dr. Dennison as the only person that he trusted.

> So when I went to the group that day—Dr. Dennison was already there—I told them it had all been an act, that the whole year and a half had been faked. And I told them how I was falling apart inside.

Nancy was livid. Dr. Dennison asked Eric to sit down in front of each member of the group and tell them one by one what he thought of them. He did. Some cried, some simply got up and left. A few stayed to tell him that he was subhuman, the lowest form of animal life. The group terminated after that day. Eric sums up this whole experience by saying "I feel encounter is destructive and humiliating."

It is significant that these methods insist on a cathartic openness and frankness, something appropriate only to a very small fraction of the population, and predictably result in their opposites: fantasy construction, lying, and a further divorce from reality, all in an attempt to please the therapist by delivering what is demanded. In this situation, the group and the therapy may be the patients' only connection with society, and they therefore often feel required to go to any lengths to prevent rejection by either because they cannot bear that isolation.

Some time during the year and a half of encounter therapy, Eric had read Janov's book, *Primal Scream*,[1] and had been completely captivated by it. When he discovered that Dr. Dennison was planning to engage in this new therapeutic activity, he immediately applied to be admitted as a patient.

Primal Scream therapy (abreactive therapy), according to the Research Task Force of the National Institute of Mental Health,[2] is

> ...designed to aid the patient to re-experience early psychological and physical hurts—in their original form. In primal therapy the release may be accompanied by

violent thrashing, screaming, and convulsive behavior, an emotional release that is believed to be curative.

The therapy is apparently based on the axiom that all neurotic behavior (later expanded by Janov to include all "mental illness") is based on an intense pain encapsulated from unhappy childhood experiences. In somewhat the same way as a boil is treated by lancing it and allowing the pus to be expressed, the act of "primalling" releases the pent up pain and tension of the earlier experiences, and results—not in relief—but in cure. As Janov puts it, "Primal patients are not acting. They *are* the little children totally out of control."

Since it happened that Dr. Dennison was now practicing primal therapy, Eric, with what little self-respect he retained, begged him to be taken on. The doctor agreed, but explained that there was a three or four month waiting list.

Primal Scream therapy was going to cost him fifteen hundred dollars, much lower than Dr. Janov's fee of $6,000. Eric "prayed every day that God would keep Dr. Dennison alive until I got into Primal Scream!" Payment was based on a twenty dollar an hour fee. Eric was eventually able to pay seven hundred dollars of his bill; he knew of another man who paid the full fifteen hundred. One girl paid nothing.

When the day came for Eric to enter therapy, a friend took him to a boarding house where the Primal Scream patients first prepared themselves. He was allowed little food or sleep there in order to experience fully the therapy that was to come. When his three weeks of "preparation" were completed he had been so broken physically and mentally that he looked gaunt and seemed estranged from the world, much as might a prisoner released from a concentration camp, a gulag.

For a therapy room, Dr. Dennison used a former lab at the university teaching hospital that had been padded partially to sound-proof it. Eric began with private sessions with Dr. Dennison. At the first session, he was told to lie down on a foam mat and "go into your feelings." After a time he was asked, "What do you feel now?" Eric felt nothing; he couldn't react. He was frozen. That night he could not sleep. At the second session, the doctor played recorded lullabies, dimmed the lights, and gave Eric a big teddy bear to play with. Once again, he lay down on the foam mat, but nothing happened. Again he was sleepless.

An hour before his third session, he conceived the notion that LSD would break down his defenses and free him to experience the "primal." After taking the drug, he felt a sensation of tremendous speed. He was on a train rushing along at four thousand miles per hour and he couldn't get off, and all around him faces came up and then evaporated. When he arrived at the therapy room, he was told to lie down as usual, but when he did the room was moving nearly as fast as the train. The doctor put on his favorite record, and dimmed the lights. Suddenly he was overwhelmed with a feeling of guilt, and a knowledge of lying and stealing.

The doctor demanded: "What did your father do?" and immediately Eric could see beatings. Did this mean his father had wanted to kill him? Had he wanted to suffocate him? As he thrashed about on the floor, Eric suddenly screamed, "No, daddy, no!" He had "primalled"!

Before the fourth session, Eric was again sleepless, so he resorted once more to LSD. Then he lay on the floor while Dr. Dennison ran slides depicting scenes of motherhood, and infancy, and cradles, and played tapes of motherly voices. He told Eric to "go into the feeling." He did, and this time he found out the basis for his intolerance of milk. Under the doctor's guidance and interpretation, he re-experienced nursing with his mother. He described it as:

> . . . an experience of great love, like the love of a man and a woman. But my parents hadn't wanted me and so my father resented my nursing. That's why my mother had to feed me quickly and half smothered me in her breast.

It was at this fourth session that the LSD Eric had used took control and he went into a drug-induced coma. Dr. Dennison apparently afraid that he might die, cradled him in his arms. Said Eric: "I came out of it with the doctor loving me, and me loving him." This event moved him profoundly and influenced many of his future actions and emotional responses. "Dr. Dennison was the only person who ever loved or cared about me. He gave himself so completely to his patients that finally he neglected his health and went into hospital."

However, at the time of Dr. Dennison's hospitalization, Eric was actually resentful of his "desertion" because he was "at the one-year-old stage." In fact, he was in such a state that he wet his pants every day. Nevertheless, he was so committed to primal therapy that, in spite of the doctor's absence, he kept "primalling on." By this time he was one of a small group whose sessions with the doctor had lasted from four in the afternoon until midnight twice a week. Now they all carried on the process of re-experiencing their lives without the doctor's help. It was a room full of people screaming "Mommy" and "Daddy," vomiting and thrashing, and worrying about whether they were having "primals" or not.

About the time the doctor returned, the group was forced to move to new quarters, because the old room became unavailable. The new room was located in a commercial district, and because it was improperly sound-proofed, there was a constant noisy exchange between the therapy group and the pool hall downstairs.

In time Eric arrived at the two-year-old level and found himself lying on his bed in his basement suite "in my own urine...in my own shit...I had become completely paranoid." One night, having decided that he had been happiest while attending university, he made up his mind to return there. He left the house at midnight, walked into the water of the lake, and began to swim toward the lights of the university in the distance. After two and a half hours in the water, his screams brought the Coast Guard to his rescue. He woke up in the emergency ward of the general hospital. He was hospitalized for four months and put on chlorpromazine, an antipsychotic drug (see Chapter 5).

When he was discharged, Dr. Dennison was there to meet him. He drove him home and then, said Eric:

> He dumped me! He told me, "Go get a job! The world doesn't owe you a living. There's no Daddy or Mommy to look after Baby Eric anymore."

Eric's discharge from the hospital was conditional on his attending a group therapy session three times a week. In this group, according to Eric, the patients "tattled" on each other.

A year later, Eric heard about the use of "nutrition and vitamins" and returned to Dr. Dennison to ask him to put him on this regimen. Dr. Dennison refused. Always the seeker, Eric found Dr. Villers through a member of the National Schizophrenia Association. Dr. Villers was an "orthomolecular psychiatrist" who indeed prescribed treatment of the kind that Eric had asked for.

The term "orthomolecular medicine" was coined by Nobel Laureate Linus Pauling to describe a form of treatment based on attempts to provide the correct internal environment in the patient's body fluids. This attempt is made by eliminating harmful substances from the diet (the definition of "harmful" varies from time to time, and from person to person), and by adding larger than customary amounts of certain vitamins and minerals. There is a growing school of physicians following this theory including a group of "orthomolecular psychiatrists" of which Dr. Villers is an exemplar. Although he does not hesitate to make use of the conventional psychotropic drugs, the mainstay of his treatment is copious use of vitamins and minerals and the removal from the diet of offending substances such as sugar, milk, wheat protein, etc. Perhaps most important is the assurance to the patient and family that the illness is biological in origin.

Mark Vonnegut has written an autobiography, *The Eden*

Express,[4] in which several years of drug-induced schizophrenia are terminated by his discovery of an orthomolecular physician, who convinced him to give up LSD and marijuana, to take suitable medication, and to take care of his nutrition and vitamin intake. According to the canons of practice of the orthomolecular psychiatrists the physician must attempt to make an accurate medical diagnosis and must relate this to the patient; this, of course, is hardly revolutionary in medicine, although it seems to us nearly so when speaking of some of the psychotherapeutic community.

Dr. Villers informed Eric that he believed him to be schizophrenic and prescribed an individualized regimen for him. Since that time, Eric has improved. He no longer takes street drugs or alcohol, no longer has the unreal feelings and experiences that characterized his participation in the varied psychotherapies, and is gradually returning to active involvement with the real world. He suffers relapses, but they are not as serious as once they were. He no longer feels that life is not worth living and looks forward to a future in which he may regain control of his former intellectual abilities and begin to use them to forge a better economic and spiritual life.

Eric is not "cured" of his illness. Schizophrenia is, in fact, at the present state of knowledge, incurable, although there is a percentage of spontaneous remissions. Attempts to cure it by "primalling," by looking back to early childhood, by inveighing against one's parents, are not only doomed to failure, but lead directly and almost inevitably to such disasters as we have recounted. Neither is it cured by "orthomolecular" treatment. As with many other chronic diseases, all we can hope to do is "manage"—render the patient's life reasonably comfortable, and as close to the quality and span of a normal person's as possible. We also have no cures for arthritis, high blood pressure, hardening of the arteries, psoriasis, or most of the diseases that afflict humanity. It is an important consideration in medical circles that one avoid either fleeing from place to place seeking out often unproved therapies or spending enormous sums to cure the incurable. Research on the causes of diseases of unknown origin, and on curative therapy for them, is obligatory, even as the physician is morally required to use in the best possible way whatever tools are available to "manage" illnesses that remain uncurable at present.

Eric's early schizophrenic symptoms led him to five long years of psychotherapy with Drs. Lake, Bailen, Isaacs, and Dennison, but in the end both he and the doctors admitted failure. It is deeply unfortunate that the various therapies tested—and the word seems well chosen—on Eric resulted only in exacerbation of his illness rather than management of it; each of these treatments failed. Only when Eric finally gave up the use of street drugs, concentrated on developing a healthful lifestyle, and met a physician who took a biological view of his problem did he slowly begin to regain his health. In addition, he joined a religious group that offered social support and an outward-reaching philosophy, which, whatever one may feel about the values of such organizations in other areas of life, has quite effectively counteracted the destructive, inward-groping psychotherapeutic treatment, and which has helped him to renew his family relationships.

Eric's experiences bring up in stark fashion the question of the value of encounter group behavior and "therapy" in "real" life. Another former encounter group member has written:

> ...much therapy is hostile, hurtful, aggressive, and destructive in the manner in which it is carried out. Patients are encouraged to be nasty and cruel to one another under the direction of the staff...The patients that do most of the attacking learn a role that is objectionable and offensive to most people outside the hospital setting. Every patient acquires this type of behavior to some degree and finds that it is unacceptable

> to people who've never been part of the psychiatric world. There have been times, to my embarrassment, that I've heard myself spouting off psychiatric put-downs that staff have used on me.

Eric summed up his own view of encounter therapy by calling it "destructive." His opinion of primal scream therapy is less conclusive. He describes it as "an attempt at a struggle—a heroic struggle." He adds, "It took the guilt trip off me, but it left me more schizophrenic than ever."

Parenthetically, we might add that the "guilt trip" was taken off Eric by transferring it to his parents. This inherent feature of many psychotherapies to provide a scapegoat, draws the condemnation of such psychiatrists as Glasser[5] and Baruk,[6] who believe that it encourages retention of an infantile mode of thinking in patients and prevents them from developing more productive modes of thought about their illness. It often poisons, perhaps permanently, the important relationship between patient and family.

Since the philosophy of Primal Therapy is to explore the pains of childhood, Eric had zeroed in on the spankings and other disciplinary measures he had received as a child, no matter that his normal brother had experienced the same upbringing. But he couldn't regress to infancy without the use of drugs, and he feels that it would be difficult for anyone to achieve what Janov had described in his book without taking street drugs before the sessions. He admits that most of his group did take drugs. Eric, of course, narrowly missed drowning in the waters of the lake; one wonders what happened to other members of the group!

The question of Eric's resort to self-administration of drugs—amphetamines at one time, LSD, alcohol later—requires a comment. During a period in history when the use of psychoactive drugs was widespread, many mentally and emotionally disturbed people looked to them as a means of gaining insight into their problems, of relieving their painful symptoms, or of transporting themselves temporarily to another, less painful world. In this deluded hope, they were encouraged by many prominent people. Timothy O'Leary was not the only university professor to advise taking this route. Some psychiatrists experimented with the use of LSD as a therapeutic agent.[3]

Whether particular psychiatrists were actively using LSD in their therapy or not, they had to be alert to the probability that their patients were taking it. Since an important part of any psychiatric interview should be detailed questioning about drug habits, and we know that Eric was taking such drugs, to his detriment, during his attendance by several psychiatrists, one can only assume either that they knew and tacitly approved, or that their history-taking was defective. What is one to make of therapies and therapists that pay so little heed to the realities of their patient's condition and the requirements of their presumed medical professionalism? In any event, Eric so idolized Dr. Dennison that the slightest threat to terminate their relationship would undoubtedly have made Eric foreswear his LSD.

In reviewing Eric's case, I contacted his younger brother, who is the principal of a high school. When I met him in his office, I was impressed at his physical resemblance to Eric—both had the same Scandinavian blonde hair and blue eyes, the same gentle manners and openness. I immediately felt at home with Karl.

My first question was about Eric's present condition. Karl informed me that he was indeed much improved. It was his impression that Dr. Villers was prescribing medication as well as orthomolecular treatment, and that this, taken with his improved life style, had made a new man of Eric. Unfortunately, the new man was not the old Eric. Although he was confident enough to be living alone in a city 2000 miles away, and was able to enter some new relationships and to go cross-country skiing, he remained unable to find a job that would utilize his university training. Karl hoped that this would come later and reported:

I met Dr. Dennison, you know. He was God to Eric. To be accepted by Dr. Dennison meant everything.

I wanted to meet this man who was so important to my brother because Eric was not doing well. I was worried about Eric because he was getting worse and worse, mentally and physically. His mental imbalance became grave, and he was physically debilitated from the improper diet and sleep deprivation that had initially been encouraged as smoothing the route to cure. So I called Dr. Dennison and it took me 2 to 3 weeks to reach him. But I did, and he came to my office and sat in the same chair where you are now.

I was shocked when I saw him. This God seemed absolutely out of control of the situation and of himself. He was intensely nervous, complained of stomach pains, and other physical symptoms.

Although I did not wish to interfere with Dr. Dennison's very important relationship with Eric, I did wish to alert Eric to the possibility of catastrophe, and predicted that Dr. Dennison was on the verge of a breakdown. Eric pooh-poohed the idea, but within a month, Dr. Dennison was in hospital, the group was disbanded, and Eric had gone for his long swim with results that I believe you already know.

I am very concerned about what happened to the group. Was Eric the only one who fell apart when it terminated abruptly? Dr. Dennison did contact Eric, although only to tell him to get lost. I hope he followed up with the remaining group members more effectively. One feels very helpless in such a situation. I would have liked to do something to insure that disaster did not overtake other members of the group but what? There is always such an air of secrecy surrounding these problems. Why can't we discuss mental illness just as easily as we discuss physical illness? Is there something shady about the illness or something shady about the practitioners?

I left feeling that if there were only fifty substantial citizens who had Karl's interest and insight, and a genuine desire to improve the lot of the mentally ill, we could begin to advance in spirit beyond the day that Dr. Philippe Pinel struck off the chains of the patients in the French mental hospital at La Bicêtre in 1793.

Where then does Primal Therapy stand? It is clear that it is very popular with some members of the public, since the Janov Institute collected some $4.2 million from 700 patients during one seven year period.[7] It has also been accepted by some members of the establishment; we have seen above that it was practiced in a university teaching hospital. Also, in a recent suit for damages by a young woman who became paraplegic after leaping from the window of a hospital to which she had been committed, the judge, in his summation, saw fit to mention that she had inadvertently witnessed a primal scream session that had intensified her fears and her desire to leave the hospital environment.

Dr. E. Fuller Torrey[8] is astounded at some of the claims made for Primal Therapy. Not only does it *cure* neuroses, psychoses, drug addiction, sexual disorders, etc., but it has been known to add an inch or more in height to a participant, to have allowed spectacles to be discarded, and to have increased both penis size and breast size (in different patients, of course). Janov says, "I think the average human today, even given all the stresses in the environment, should live beyond 100 years. The way to achieve all this, I submit, is Primal Therapy. This is neither esoteric theorizing, Utopian daydreaming, nor guess-work. Our research at the Primal Laboratory appears to make increased longevity quite possible." As Torrey suggests, $6000 is a modest fee for such benefits.

Unfortunately, the research that Dr. Janov quotes proves nothing about longevity, if indeed it proves anything at all. It has been done in his laboratory on 22 subjects and has not been verified by an independent and objective laboratory. The measurements made were routine vital signs such as pulse, blood pressure, and electroencephalograph tracings. Although

Janov states there were controls, he has not published his findings on them. There are no statistics, and therefore, considering the short life span of the Primal Laboratory, there could be none demonstrating that patients who had undergone the treatment lived longer than people who had not.

At any rate, I am not primarily concerned with the efficacy of Primal Therapy as used on voluntary patients who are prepared to pay a small fortune for its application to them. (One of the criteria the FDA applies in deciding whether to allow the use and sale of medications, clinical apparatus, and laboratory equipment is that they should be efficacious for the purposes claimed. Somehow this principle has not yet been applied to the marketing of such nonmaterial processes as systems of therapy.) My primary concern here is with the deleterious effects of a system that requires the patients to fast, be deprived of sleep, to dwell on real or imagined childhood pains, to writhe and scream and vomit, and to destroy the deepest feelings of trust and respect among families.

Torrey states that Janov accepts some schizophrenics (as Dr. Dennison did Eric) and that some schizophrenics undergoing Primal Therapy may get worse (as did Eric). In addition, "Intense abreactions may also precipitate suicidal impulses..." It seems strange that a product with all this potential for harm is allowed to be marketed at high prices without the usual demonstration of efficacy for the purpose claimed and relative freedom from harmful side effects.

A psychiatrist who practiced Primal Scream therapy explained in a recent lecture that he insisted on his patients being isolated for three weeks from everything.

> This is so that my patient cannot escape the painful parts of his past experience—I focus on what is happening inside of them, and I look at the patient's own defenses when dealing with pain....Medication is not really useful if the patient opened up and expressed his feelings....I

> must bring forth from the unconscious the memory and affect of repressed material... cure is the memory of the event....I want my patients to talk not *about* their parents, but *to* their parents.

According to the NIMH report of 1975,[9] "no systematic independent research has assessed the validity... [of a therapy] that makes use of violent thrashing, convulsive behavior and screaming. I can find no later answer to this question. In addition, there are no clinical results published by independent psychiatrists using primal scream therapy. One can only guess, therefore, at the casualty rate among Primal Scream patients, although Dr. Lowy of the University of Toronto declares: "There *are* demonstrated cases hurt by abreactive (primal scream) therapy."

It is sad that a such large industry is based on holding out futile hopes of cure to one of the most unhappy segments of our society. The public is alert to such abuses when they entail physical products, such as medication. There have been prosecutions of physicians and others who persisted in using cancer drugs after they had been declared inefficacious by the FDA. There have also been prosecutions of lay practitioners of acupuncture, presumably because they were practicing medicine without a license. There is a very fine point between the physical manipulation of a patient in acupuncture by a non-MD and the physical deprivations that go along with the psychological manipulations of Primal Therapy, also frequently practiced by non-MDs. In my opinion, the potential for harm by unproved fads in psychotherapy is far greater than that possible with acupuncture or laetrile.

It would appear that no one is prepared to demand scientific verification from the proponents of all too many psychotherapies, demands that are made routinely when treatment of a bodily ill is in question. We seem to be dealing with the ancient mind-body duality, a view that makes treatment of the mind more a matter of religion or faith than of science, and therefore immune to the controls we demand of normal medical treatment.

My hope is that we are on the verge of breaking down the effects of the mind–body duality. With the recognition that the mind is the mode of action of one of the largest and most active organs in the body should come the demand that more, rather than less, scientific rigor be required of claims for understanding the mechanisms of and treatments for this system in which are concentrated all the joys and sorrows of human existence.

4

The Mystery of Lithium

At the time this case study was made, Gary Findley was thirty-three years old. He is the middle child in a family of three. His older sister is a teacher, happily married with a young family; his younger brother earned his master's degree in chemistry, is now in charge of the lab for a large processing company, and is happily married. Their father was in the armed forces overseas when Gary was born and as a result didn't meet the boy until he was two years old, when he returned to civilian life as a professor of geography at a state university. When Gary was twenty-eight, his father died. Even before her husband's death, Ms. Findley had worked part-time in a baby clinic, and since his death, she has lived alone, but is very active socially, and still works part time.

When interviewed, Gary began:

> It is only since I got medication from Dr. Edmunds that I can look back and pinpoint the time when my troubles started. I realize now that I first became depressed when I was fourteen. I imagine my body chemistry was changing and it just took a wrong turn somewhere. In the last semester of Grade 12 and on into my first attempt at university, I began to drink quite heavily and to feel lonely and isolated from my friends. I developed new friends, of course, but they were what I would call—well, a lower order of friends.
>
> *Question:* Which came first—the drinking or the feelings of loneliness?

Gary: Well, I first started drinking very casually when I was fifteen and it made me feel really elated and happy. When I wasn't drinking I felt very much down, so I suppose I was using this as a way to lift myself out of my gloom. Of course at the time I didn't think of it that way; I just thought of it as having a good time. I was able to do things that I guess most people are able to do without artificial chemical changes. I began to smoke at the age of fifteen, too. A pack a day. And from then on I never smoked less than that.

By the time I was twenty I was drinking heavily every night and smoking at least three packs a day. I had dropped out of university, and had taken a job washing pots in one of the university cafeterias. I realized that something was definitely wrong, but I was twenty-three before I made an effort to do something about it. Then I went to our family doctor and he referred me to a psychiatrist in the city. But Dr. Simon just rubbed me the wrong way. He insisted that I had been programmed for university by my parents, although I argued that it had been my own idea. After that he wanted to start digging around in my childhood. I thought: Well, this is a load of crap! And I went back to my old ways again.

I had become obese by then, though I'd never been fat as a child. My weight had gone up from about one hundred seventy pounds to about two hundred and forty. I was smoking four packs a day and literally drinking thirty or forty glasses of beer every night! Then I started smoking marijuana and hashish. I held various jobs in construction, but eventually wound up back in town working as a teamster driving a forklift.

That was about five years ago, and it marked the point when I really decided things had to change. I quit smoking then, and almost three years ago now, after considerable turmoil and difficulty, I quit drinking entirely, and I quit smoking the various cannabis drugs. I actually hadn't enjoyed drinking or smoking dope for a good solid year before I quit, and I'd always said that as soon as I stopped enjoying it, I'd quit. I haven't had either of them since. Once I did try smoking marijuana later on, but I hated it. I just had no interest in it anymore.

But it was after I'd cut these things out that I became really depressed, though I wouldn't go back to them because I just damn well vowed that I wasn't going to wind up like the people you see down on Skid Row.

Question: Can you describe the nature of your depression?

Gary: Well, in the period before I'd quit drinking, I'd considered suicide at various times. I went so far as getting razor blades out at two o'clock one morning. I must have made some noise, some cry of despair, I guess—or maybe I even called out to my mother, because she came in and took them away from me.

Actually, I had thought about suicide fairly often, but it was usually in pretty abstract terms. I considered seeing another psychiatrist, but frankly I didn't trust them because I'd heard so many crackpot psychoanalytic or psychiatric theories rolling around. I just wasn't really interested, so I put it off. But about six or seven months after I had quit my chemical dependencies, I did go to see a psychiatrist because I realized I was feeling really suicidal. Dr. Moraine tried to point out alternative ways of living. He told me that I didn't have to go to university, and that nobody was holding a gun to my head to make me drive a forklift.

Since I'd read about the use of lithium for depression, I asked him to prescribe it for me. "Oh no, that's not for you," he told me. Instead he put me on Mellaril, which did help me, because it sort of tranquilized me, and made me feel optimistic for a few months.

Question: What dosage were you on?

Gary: Dr. Moraine made it just the minimum dosage—thirty milligrams—and when that didn't do anything I started taking fifty, which was still very mild, but at least it was helpful for about three months. For the next four or

five months I just went to see him once a week to talk.
Question: What did you talk about?
Gary: Well, he'd just sit there and pull on his pipe, and we'd chat away. I guess I was waiting for some positive counselling, some reason for going on, but the whole thing petered out after about eight months. He told me then that there really wasn't much more we could do right then. He said maybe as time went by I might want to see him again, and if I did, I should certainly call him. But he said that things had pretty well run their course between us.
Question: Were you given a prescription for continuing medication?
Gary: No. I just went back to my old ways of coping with things, until about eight months after I stopped seeing Dr. Moraine when I enrolled—volunteered, I guess—to be part of Dr. Campbell's depression study program at the university. By chance, out of the four different therapies being used, I drew behavior modification. My therapist was a very supportive person, a Mormon. She's not a physician, she's a clinical psychologist with a good background in social psychology. She was very helpful in many ways, but nonetheless after about three sessions with her I guess I sort of relaxed mentally and the bottom fell out. I slid into a really deep depression. I'd been thoroughly depressed all winter, ever since I'd left Dr. Moraine, and I guess I'd come to the point where I wasn't able to hold myself up anymore. And I didn't see any point in trying because I felt that the program wasn't helping me. I became very suicidal, but on the night that I decided that I couldn't cope any longer, I also had to attend a therapy session. So I went, and then I told her that I was planning to go off the bridge. She phoned Dr. Campbell and told him that I was feeling this way, and they discussed whether or not I should be admitted to hospital. But they left the decision up to me. It was pretty obvious, though, that they didn't think I should.
Question: What gave you that impression?

Gary: I'd talked to the clinical psychologist in the next office, and she'd told me that they all thought that the hospital just dragged people in there, doped them up and fattened them up, but that they didn't accomplish much. They might actually keep me from jumping off the bridge that night, but they couldn't give me any long-term therapy. And you know, they don't just claim to do crisis management there; they really claim to do long term therapy. And they don't. It was just luck that I didn't jump off the bridge that night.

Question: Did you leave Dr. Campbell's program at that time?

Gary: No. Dr. Campbell and my therapist decided that they could give me a little Valium to calm my anxiety, if not my depression, without invalidating the behavior modification side of the program as it were. I went on seeing my therapist until the twelve week program was finished, and when it ended in July I felt better—somewhat better. So I enrolled in college, but toward the end of September, I started to slide back down into another depression, and I could feel that it was shaping up to be a bad one. October was really difficult; I was able to do almost no school work.

But sometime during that month I heard of a psychiatrist who believed in prescribing medication for serious depression. Our family doctor arranged an appointment in early November with Dr. Edmunds. I liked him right away, and I had confidence in him because it was obvious he had complete confidence in his own ability. It didn't take him long to decide that my depression had a biological base and could be managed with medication in the same way that diabetes and high blood pressure can be managed. He hospitalized me, and put me on antidepressants and lithium. It was a little rough to become accustomed to for the first week or so, but since then things have been vastly improved, although I still see Dr. Edmunds periodically. Now my school work is going well. Instead of being forced to drop out, I had four A's and a B last term, which is remarkable for somebody who's been out of school for fifteen years, don't you think? I wouldn't have achieved those marks if it hadn't been for the medication, for the lift I get from taking the antidepressants. Of course, it's not just the lift—its the relief from depression, and it's totally different from anything I had experienced previously.

If it hadn't been for this medication, for its lifting of this great internal cloud of heavy doubt and worry—everything that goes with depression and anxiety—I wouldn't even know how long I'd been depressed. It's as if I were a fish being pulled out of water; I hadn't even known I was in that water until I was pulled out, and that's the way I continue to feel about it.

Question: The last time we talked, Gary, you spoke of law school. Are you still considering this?

Gary: Oh yes. Just now at the college I am actually enrolled in a two-year program, but the director of the program has suggested that I write the entrance exams for law school in April. He himself is absolutely certain that I'll pass them, so I might well be enrolled in law school next fall.

Question: Gary, what effect did your illness have on your family?

Gary: Well, my dad never had much liking for psychiatrists at all, although he was dead by the time I was suffering from the worst of it. Then, too, my mother carried a double burden of guilt. She felt just terrible, you know, thinking: "What have we done to blight his life? Why is he so depressed and suicidal? Could we have been better parents?" Of course, she looked back on the mistakes that they had made and the troubles that they had had and thought: "My god, here's how we have ruined Gary's life." But it's worth pointing out that I have an older sister and a younger brother who turned out fine. They grew up in the same environment that I did, but since they just didn't develop the same problems, I don't really believe that any blame for what's happened to me accrues to my parents. I continue to have a wonderful friendship with my mother.

On the other hand, Gary's mother definitely does fault herself for her shortcomings and failures, and continually questions herself even now about the consequences of her role in his life. She asks herself the questions most reasonably educated, concerned parents might ask: Did Gary's troubles stem from the fact that his father was in the army during his early life? Was this compounded by his displacement as the center of attention when his younger brother was born? Why were his sister and brother normal happy individuals? What did I do to cause Gary to be depressed?

When interviewed she told of an incident that Gary had omitted from his story:

> It happened while Gary was seeing Dr. Moraine. One night I found him in his room with tears rolling down his face. I sat down and talked gently to him and he told me then that he'd decided to jump off the bridge. I tried to convince him it wouldn't solve anything and then we just sat there and talked together into the night until he felt somewhat calmer.
>
> You know, I'd never interfered when Gary decided to go to a psychiatrist for help—I'd been glad, of course, but that was his affair. But that night I phoned Dr. Moraine to tell him what Gary planned to do, that he had the place picked out and everything.
>
> *Question:* How did the doctor react?
>
> *Ms. Findley:* He told me he'd just have to tell Gary everything I'd said about him in my phone call. He had just assumed there was an adversary relationship between Gary and me. So I just said, You go right ahead and tell him! But for goodness sake, do something for him!

Gary's adventures with "behavior modification" therapy in Dr. Campbell's program began with an assessment of his academic and social aspirations. The goal of the therapy was to change behavior that the therapist considered destructive into behavior constructive to his aspirations. The therapist decided that Gary's first positive move must be a return to his long-abandoned university career. He was therefore told to bring his registration forms to the next therapy session. He actually did this, but unfortunately it coincided with the day that "the bottom fell out."

Despite the doctor's theory and description of the program, Gary's treatment can scarcely be called behavior modification, the *sine qua non* of which is not an attempt to modify behavior (indeed, this is the purpose of *all* therapy, including drug therapy), but the manner in which the attempt is made. Behavior modification therapy, based on the richly productive work of Pavlov, B. F. Skinner, and others over many decades, assumes that maladaptive behavior is the result of conditioning, and that the route to change is to de-condition the subject, using the classical modalities of aversion, reward, reinforcement, and so on. There was no evidence of any use of these techniques in the course of Gary's treatment, and we must therefore assume that some error has been made in the doctor's own label for this phase of Gary's treatment.

Because he happens to be a voracious reader, Gary struck us as one of the more fortunate sufferers of depression. He knew that antidepressants existed because he had read about them, but he had been required first to undergo long courses of pointless and often destructive psychotherapy, treatment that almost resulted in his suicide, before he found a doctor who would prescribe this medicine that he so desperately needed.

Many incidents in the case of Carol Winfield resemble Gary's problems. A homemaker, Carol did some volunteer work, and had a full social life. Her husband was a successful lawyer, and her three sons were thriving adolescents.

She was about forty when she became depressed. She tried initially to ignore the symptoms on the theory that they were transient. When at last she realized that her problems were not improving, that her condition was worsening, she went to see a psychiatrist. A year of one-to-one therapy saw no improvement, and in fact she now felt completely worthless and was considering suicide. In desperation, she left her family and went to a distant city where she voluntarily hospitalized herself. Here she received further individual therapy and was eventually introduced into group therapy.

Later she said, "I was accused of acting as a mother figure in the group sessions because I tried to protect people. Sometimes, you see, they'd keep at one of the group until that person broke down, and to me that was just plain destructive. Then they'd ask me, 'Why do you protect him? Why the mother role?' "

But the therapists' efforts to improve Carol's own welfare were centered on her relationship with her husband. They were determined to involve him also in therapy sessions, but he refused. He could see nothing in his relationship with his wife that might have caused her illness. The therapists, therefore, pointing at his refusal to help, encouraged Carol to find her own apartment and to retrain for a new career as a medical librarian. She had actually begun the search for an apartment and enrolled in a hospital training program for some brush-up courses when her depression began spontaneously to lift and she realized how much she missed her family. She returned to her home town and went into hospital there. Not long after, a friend visited her and told her about antidepressants. Carol located a psychiatrist who was indeed willing to prescribe medication rather than group therapy for her depression. After trials with several antidepressants and lithium, Carol's periods of depression became fewer, and she leveled off on lithium and other medication.

Helen Sealem, at forty-three, realized that the "moods" she had been experiencing since childhood had now become enormous problems. Her normal state was tremendously energetic and creative. She could do three people's work without feeling fatigue; but then periods of black depression would close in on her; she could not bear to get out of bed, or leave the house, and she became afraid of people, and convinced of her own worthlessness. Yet Helen said her external life could not have been better: a divorcee, she was involved in a comfortable liaison. She was pursuing a very successful career, and her grown children, with whom she enjoyed a very close relationship, were involved in their own careers, and not making emotional demands on her. Why, then, was she experiencing these terrible depressions? For two years she suffered, dreading the long years of psychoanalysis that she thought would be needed to uncover the roots of her problems. But when her problems proved no longer bearable, she finally went to a psychiatrist. On her first visit, he took great care to consider whether there was possibly a biological problem underlying her illness, and apparently deciding that there was, spoke about lithium. She learned that the drug might be a nearly complete answer to her depressions, ultimately. Within weeks she had returned to a wholly normal existence. Her drama classes came to life. She could demonstrate pathos, joy, and spontaneity to her students. Her frozen emotions had thawed.

Helen's is very nearly a classical manic–depressive case. Her ability to persist in almost superhuman efforts is a characteristic that verges on the hypomanic, except that hers had always before been under control. This type of borderline-controlled hypomania probably characterizes many public figures who can survive on four hours of sleep, or without vacations for years. Then, as Winston Churchill said, "The black dog" gets them.

It is probably the sub-manic element in Helen's depression that made her react so dramatically and effectively to lithium. As will be explained later in this book, the manic-depressive is the greatest beneficiary of lithium, even when the symptoms are purely depressive. It must be remembered, of course, that few patients respond so rapidly or dramatically as Helen did to lithium.

One can find in syndicated columns in the newspaper, popular magazines, and TV and radio programs, personal accounts of individuals who hope that their experience with medication will encourage others who fear treatment for their illnesses. Tony Orlando, colorfully, if not too accurately, describes his hyperactivity and depression as "a breakdown in a person's cell structure." Orlando is a manic-depressive, "like Abraham Lincoln, and Winston Churchill and Theodore Roosevelt and perhaps thousands of others who never understood the disease that was making them ill."

Orlando could move with amazing energy. He was a successful performer until, without warning, he would slump into depression. The management of his illness began when he heard a program discussing Dr. Ronald R. Fieve's book on manic-depressive illness, phoned Dr. Fieve, the author of *Moodswing*,[1] and eventually obtained treatment with lithium.

The public learned more about manic-depressives when the popular TV character "Maude" let it be known that she was a manic-depressive on medication. Vivian Leigh, too, star of *Gone With the Wind*, battled attacks of this illness for years. She was protected from publicity by friends who thought that public knowledge of it might damage her career. But, thankfully, we have advanced since Leigh's time. Joshua Logan, director and producer, announced that lithium makes it possible for him to continue his career.

Sidney Katz,[2] Canadian medical journalist, was asked whether lithium may be the answer for alcoholics. He cited research[3] that showed that 75% of *depressed* alcoholics became teetotallers when treated with lithium, whereas the untreated patients increased their alcohol intake. None of the members of a control group taking dummy pills exactly resembling lithium were found to drink less. Katz concludes that the use of lithium carbonate is one of the great therapeutic advances in medicine in the past decade.

The National Institute of Mental Health report[4] agrees. "Unipolar and bipolar patients (depressives and manic-depressives) can now be treated with lithium carbonate, use of which may become as significant a development as use of insulin for diabetes."

Lest it be thought that lithium is a panacea, with the near certainty of helping many people suffering from a broad diversity of problems, a drug with practically no potential for harm, we must observe at this point the reverse side of the lithium coin.

In the first place, although there is no question that lithium is virtually specific in shortening dramatically the acute, manic stage of bipolar (manic-depressive) disease, the certainty of its value decreases as we descend to the depressed phase of the illness, and even more as its use is considered in prophylaxis. As it happens, the most important potential use of lithium would initially appear to be in the prevention or mitigation of unipolar depression, a common disorder in comparison with the rarity of manic-depressive disease. But although many physicians are confident[5] that lithium is helpful in this application, it is precisely here that the greatest doubts of its efficacy arise.

There would be no problem in taking a chance with the uncertain efficacy if the drug were harmless. Unfortunately, evidence is accumulating that this may not be true. Lithium salts exhibit two kinds of toxicity—acute, resulting from overdosage, and chronic, owing to prolonged administration at levels that do not cause acute intoxication.

Many physicians are concerned solely about the acute effects and monitor their patients' blood levels quite frequently. They are probably concentrating on the wrong problem. Although lithium intoxication can be severe and even lead to the death of the patient, it is rare, with only 123 cases having been reported in the literature through 1977.[6] Most of the patients who grew very ill had been showing signs of toxicity—tremors, weakness, rigidity, diarrhea—for days. Had they been followed closely, or been taught to report symptoms, a serum lithium concentration determination at the time symptoms commenced would usually have shown elevated values and stopping the lithium dosages at that time would have reversed the intoxication.

When a lithium intoxication is allowed to proceed for days or weeks, the patient's kidney function becomes impaired, and even stopping the lithium may not reduce either the amount of lithium in the body or the symptoms. Such patients may require hemodialysis—use of the artificial kidney—to rid them of their excess lithium. In any event, if patients are observed carefully and treated at the first signs of intoxication, or even if they become more severely affected but eventually come to successful treatment, they recover completely. Of the 123 patients reported ill in the major study, only two died.

Perhaps more important can be the insidious effects of long-term lithium ingestion at normal therapeutic levels. Although it has long been known[7] that patients (and laboratory animals) given lithium become thirsty and pass large quantities of urine, it is only in the last five years that research has demonstrated that there are two processes occurring. The first is a reversible effect that occurs only while the lithium is being ingested, and is therefore of no long term concern. However, it is unfortunate that patients who may be taking other drugs causing dry mouth also suffer excessive water loss in the urine from taking lithium, and therefore have a second reason for consuming large amounts of water. The more serious lithium-related problem is that permanent damage to the kidneys of a type that causes increased urinary output after the lithium is discontinued appears to be possible. Biopsies of the kidneys of such patients[8] have shown scarring, which must be irreversible. What is not known as yet is how extensive the scarring can be, how much of kidney *function* is recoverable if lithium is withdrawn, what is the relationship between dosage and duration of medication on the one hand,

and kidney damage on the other. Scarring occurs with age in everyone, but not to the extent shown by patients on long-term lithium.

The problem is not unique to lithium or indeed to psychotropic drugs. There are virtually no drugs without some deleterious side effects. It becomes a matter of judgment, for physician and patient alike, to decide whether the cure is worse than the disease. The decision in some cases of mental illness may actually reduce to one of whether it is desirable to live a long life that is not worth living (or which is perhaps terminated by suicide) or a shorter but happier one.

Such a decision is an easy one when dealing with acute mania. In the first place, the drug is specific, and therefore justifies the risk of its use. Secondly, it need only be taken for a short time to control the mania, and the risk of permanent damage under these conditions is negligible.

The problem arises most seriously, however, when prophylactic use of lithium is considered. Here the benefits are not so clearly marked and the risks are greater. The history of the patient must be taken into account when attempting to estimate whether yet another risk can be taken—that being the risk of leaving patients unmedicated until their symptoms reappear in the hope that treatment can later be instituted before it becomes too difficult, or before the patients do themselves some serious harm.

At the outpatient schizophrenic clinic of the Clarke Institute of Psychiatry,[9] a very reasonable approach has been taken to the related problem of the long term toxicity of phenothiazines. These drugs are at the present moment essential to the successful management of schizophrenia, but also have the potential to cause a serious long-term side effect—tardive dyskinesia (see Chapter 2)—that may also become irreversible. Although there is no question that the incidence of relapse into schizophrenia is very closely related to withdrawal of the drug, the Clarke Institute protocol calls for intermittent phenothiazine holidays of about six weeks duration. The patient is kept under more careful observation during this period, and medication is reinstituted as soon as the early symptoms of the underlying schizophrenia reappear. The resultant decrease in total drug exposure, together with its intermittency, is expected to reduce the incidence of tardive dyskinesia. Regrettably, such a regimen cannot be applied to patients who do not report regularly for assessment, or who rapidly relapse into a flagrant psychosis that is then resistant to treatment. In such patients, the correct decision is probably to accept the risk of drug side effects in order to avoid the virtual certainty of prolonged or even permanent hospitalization.

So we come back to some of the oldest wisdom of medicine. We cure rarely. We must weigh the pros and cons of every treatment and, with the concurrence of the patient, do our best to manage as successfully as possible.

5

The Biology of Mental Illness

We have been extremely interested thus far in presenting the cases of victims of mental disease, people who, although previously normal, became utterly incapable of coping with their jobs, their families, their social relationships, or even their own nutrition. Some came to perceive the world in terms quite unlike the perceptions of the rest of the population, some became unable to leave their beds or their homes, and some attempted or actually committed suicide. All of them spent years trying to recover some semblance of their former personalities.

In spite of years of research and enormous expense, medical science still has much to learn about the fundamental pathology, cause, and treatment of diseases of many of the human organ systems. It is not so surprising, therefore, that this is also true of diseases of one of the largest, most complex, and most energy-consuming organs—the brain. However, there are enough facts and probable truths known about the brain to supply a measure of guidance to those who treat brain diseases, and to those who must live with such diseases, either in themselves or in someone close to them.

The first problem to be faced is the lack of a generally agreed-upon definition of mental disease. Neither in the lay mind nor in psychiatric literature has there been a clear distinction between serious and even life-threatening diseases, such as schizophrenia and depression on the one hand, and forms of behavior that do not fulfill any medical criteria of disease, such as homosexuality and social deviance, on the other. It is as if medicine were to suggest that cancer of the spine and bad posture were to be considered more or less as variants of the same condition, namely spinal inadequacy. Incapacitating mental conditions that afflict a certain percent of the population must be taken as seriously as—or, because of the additional anguish, more seriously than—heart disease, cancer, or stroke.

Although there is a compendium of mental disease, the American Psychiatric Association's *Diagnostic and Statistical Manual* (DSM),[1] it has hitherto been a catalog of miscellaneous conditions having the common feature of mental symptoms. Interestingly, the first philosophical analysis of this manual was precipitated in 1973[2] by a proposal to delete homosexuality from the psychiatric nomenclature. Having achieved this *tour de force,* the APA has set up a task force under the chairmanship of R. L. Spitzer* to present to the Society a proposed definition of mental illness in order to provide a rationale for the inclusion or exclusion of specific illnesses. This task force is having stormy sailing, with objections being raised not only to specific wording and concepts of the definition of mental disorder, and of illness in general, but also to the entire proposal to produce a general definition of mental illness. Spitzer is apparently proposing that neuroses—the milder psychological deviations that were the entire subject matter of a century of Freudian theory and practice—be deleted from DSM-III. It remains to be seen whether this proposal will be accepted.

What we consider mental diseases in this book are conditions that involve a complete change from normal behavior. There are two possible reasons for such changes. The first one, known as the biogenic theory, postulates that some serious malfunction has occurred in the brain. The second, the psychogenic theory, argues that psychological stresses, new or

*No relation to the present authors.

old, have caused a behavior change. The cases we recount here demonstrate clearly that the second hypothesis can have only limited validity, not only because these patients had suffered no greater psychological trauma than the majority of the population, but also because they either failed to improve when treated with psychotherapy, or when they did show improvement, it was more closely related to the use of suitable medication than to psychological manipulation.

Upon being shown this argument, an internist friend argued that the reasoning was partly specious. "It is a well-known fact that people display a wide variety of different responses to the same stimuli. It does not strain one's credulity to believe that, in some people, serious mental illness can follow serious personal, domestic, and vocational problems with which a person cannot cope." Which is precisely what we have stated. If one person, suffering from a surfeit of such personal difficulties, proves able to cope and goes on strengthened by the experience, while a second becomes mentally ill, what can be the difference between the two? Temperament? Inner strength? Individual variation? Are not all these poetic expressions for the biological variability that we assert is the basis of serious mental disease.

But there are far more cogent arguments than the philosophical for asserting that the two main mental illnesses—schizophrenias and manic-depressive (bipolar) disease—are biological.

First is the genetic evidence. It has been known for a long while that the incidence of mental diseases in close relatives of patients exceeds the general incidence in its general population by a factor of about 10. It has been argued that this does not prove genetic transmittance because it could be the similar environment and upbringing of siblings (who, however, are not always or mostly involved in the excess incidence) that was responsible. This argument has been definitively settled by a number of studies, prominently those of Seymour Kety[3,4] and his coworkers who traced the fates of identical twins who had been adopted out of their families of birth at an early age. The twins, then, with the same biological inheritance, had very different environments from infancy. The result was a high degree of concordance in the development of schizophrenia among the twins with few, if any, of the other foster children in the same homes developing the disease.

Again, different classes of patients respond very differently to the same drug. Use of imipramine, a tricyclic antidepressant (see below), leads to marked improvement in mood and motor activity in depressed patients, has no psychological effect on normal people, and induces a significant activation of psychotic symptoms in schizophrenics. Similar effects are obtained with other drugs, both of a type used in psychopharmacology and other sorts. We are, in fact, approaching the time when an individual's response to drugs will be of greater use in making psychiatric diagnoses than the conventional subjective analyses that are now being used.

Not only do the psychological effects of drugs vary with the patient's disease, but so also do some physical parameters. In a rather hazardous experiment, DFP, an organic phosphate anticholinesterase (related to the drug physostigmine and some of the more potent insecticides),[5] was administered for seven days to schizophrenics, manic-depressives, and normals. Almost all of the manic-depressives experienced a fall in blood pressure that lasted for a week after the withdrawal of the drug. No schizophrenic patient showed a fall, and there was, on the contrary, a tendency for the blood pressure to rise. The schizophrenic patients also showed a remarkably low incidence of so-called "muscarinic" side effects of the drug, again indicating a biological difference between the two groups of patients. Mentally, the bipolar group, if they showed any effect, tended to become depressed, as did the normal group. One third of the schizophrenics showed a severe activation of schizophrenic symptoms, an effect noticed with none of the other groups.

An interesting argument in favor of the biogenic theory is

that a large variety of distinctly physical diseases can cause symptoms that mimic "functional" mental illnesses such as schizophrenia and depression. Some of the diseases that have been the occasion of admissions to mental hospitals include brain tumors, hypo- or hyperthyroidism, pernicious anemia, diabetes mellitus, islet cell tumor of the pancreas, senile or presenile dementia, pellagra, uremia, porphyria, and chemical intoxication. That such a wide variety of physical or chemical causes can result in mental disorders suggests that most serious mental diseases will ultimately be proved to have been caused by biological or chemical malfunction.

The term "functional" needs some discussion. Diseases are roughly divided into anatomical and functional. Those diseases with an anatomic basis, such as a missing leg, cirrhosis of the liver, or an infected lung, can be seen with the naked eye or with the aid of a microscope. However, it is the functional element that is really at issue: the amputee cannot walk properly, the cirrhotic loses many functions of a healthy liver, such as the ability to excrete bile and avoid jaundice, or the ability to synthesize certain necessary proteins, so that is is really the impaired function that is the problem, not necessarily the impaired anatomic structure. A cauliflower ear, of course, may be considered an anatomical impairment, but it cannot be considered to be a disease since no impairment in function occurs.

The other category of diseases is functional. These diseases cause impairment in function without known anatomical (or, by extension, chemical) impairment. There is, however, another possible interpretation of the term "functional," that is, that the anatomical, microanatomical, or biochemical basis of the disease is *not yet known.* For example, there was a time not much over a century ago when the victims of diabetes mellitus were known to have markedly impaired function—they ate ravenously but lost weight, drank copiously and poured out equally copious amounts of urine (giving rise to half the name: diabetes = a running trough). No anatomic impairment in these patients could be demonstrated until they had suffered from the disease for decades. The only known abnormality was the seemingly irrelvant fact that the urine was sweet (mellitus = honey-like). So diabetes was a functional disorder until more and more refined measurements ultimately showed that the ability to control sugar metabolism was grossly impaired because the patient's pancreas did not secrete a vital hormone known as insulin. Why the pancreas is defective is still not known, and since the defect cannot be anatomically demonstrated, the disease evidently occurs at the cellular and biochemical, rather than the organ, level. Thus diabetes is no longer included in the category of functional diseases, because so much more of its pathological and physiological basis is now understood.

A much rarer disease, called familial periodic paralysis, has an even more dramatic history. In this disease, which tends to afflict more than one member of a family, the patient is apparently healthy to all physical, chemical, and X-ray investigation, at least to all that was available fifty years ago. Suddenly, with no apparent precipitating cause, the patient develops a profound paralysis, just as some hysterics are purported to do. Then just as suddenly the same patient recovers to a thoroughly normal state of health. Aside from the flaccidity of the muscles during the attack, no physical or chemical abnormality could be found.

But about forty years ago, a new instrument, the flame photometer, entered the hospital laboratory, enabling routine measurement to be made of serum potassium and sodium. It was already known that these inorganic ions were involved in nerve conduction, and it was consequently natural to measure their concentration in the blood of sufferers from familial periodic paralysis. Not surprisingly, it was found that the patient's normal level of serum potassium dropped precipitously into a range compatible with paralysis just before an attack and returned to normal as the attack terminated. Although we do not know the reason for these changes in the level of serum potassium, we now understand them as the reason for the paralysis, and can rename the disease as familial intermittent hypokalemia, to use a little medical jargon, because hypokalemia means low blood potassium. The label now indicates the cause rather than the symptom, and we have eliminated another "functional" illness from the list of unexplained diseases.

In the field of psychiatry, the most important diseases still fall in this "functional" category, but because the symptoms of the diseases are mental rather than physical, the term "functional" tends to imply that the *cause* as well as the symptoms are mental, that there is no underlying physical basis, and that the patients are responsible in some semivoluntary way for their own diseases. The connotation is somewhat similar to that of the words "psychosomatic" and "psychogenic."

In addition to meaning that the cause of a disease is unknown, the term "functional" is too often used to mean "I don't know the cause," although it may be one that is well recognized. It is shown in Chapter 7 that approximately 10% of all patients who are referred to psychiatric clinics—presumably for "functional" illness, since this is the major category dealt with in such clinics—are in fact suffering from a clear physical illness that alone is sufficient to account for the psychiatric symptoms.

Perhaps the argument up to this point is well summarized by a principle enunciated by Sir Isaac Newton in the early 18th century: great effects demand great causes. With this in mind, one's credulity is strained to accept the idea that such serious symptoms as loss of drive and the ability to plan ahead, inability to take a job or keep friends, prolonged loss of contact with reality, and even suicide could arise from such common and easily adapted-to events as family disagreements, improper upbringing, etc. Indeed, who *is* properly brought up, and who sets the standards for proper child nurture from one generation to the next?

It seems more reasonable in the light of the histories of diabetes and familial periodic paralysis we have just examined, to believe that a disease such as schizophrenia is a "functional" disease that is only waiting for its category to be changed; for it can be only a matter of time before medical scientists develop some powerful new methods to measure the abnormal chemical constituents in the central nervous system. Thus it seems willfully shortsighted to persist in designating schizophrenia as a self-caused psychological aberration (see Chapter 8).

Are there any examples of mental diseases moving from the category of "functional" to partially or completely understood entities. No, not in the sense that diabetes and familial periodic paralysis are now so understood, but there are beginnings.

According to psychogenic theories of disease, the external social and interpersonal influences to which a person has been subjected should correlate with the onset of disease. Advocates of these theories claim to have made such correlations. The difficulty is that each author correlates these diseases with different phenomena: for example, improper toilet training, a cold mother, an overprotective mother, the death of a loved one, or some combination of these. But the correlations are retrospective—that is, attributed after the patient has become ill. And they are usually not controlled—that is, no comparison is made with the proportion of the normal population exposed to the same influences.

In the past, the idea that major psychoses were psychosocially caused was given support by one of the classics of anthropological literature—Ruth Benedict's[6] *Patterns of Culture*. This landmark of cultural relativity presented a persuasive argument that virtually all human behavior—

including the psychotic—was culturally conditioned, and that behavior that would be considered psychotic in one society might be considered valuable and superior in another. One of her outstanding examples was the shaman in Siberian tribes who, although clearly psychotic by Ms. Benedict's standards, was a valuable and respected member of society. These conclusions from *Patterns of Culture* have been accepted uncritically until recently, when a new generation of anthropologists has reinvestigated the problem with a more powerful methodology than that used by Benedict. The conclusions reached by Dr. Jane Murphy[7] are almost diametrically opposed. Using two relatively primitive groups who were as culturally separated as could be found—a group of Siberian Eskimos living on an island in the Bering Strait, and a group of Yorubas living in Nigeria—she actually obtained consensus among the groups not only about the meaning and symptomatology of "crazy," but also about who in these groups could be so described. In the first place, she found the described symptomatology to agree within the two groups, and also to agree well with our concept of psychotic or even schizophrenic behavior. When describing illnesses "not of the flesh and bones" both groups talked about "getting wild . . . going out of her mind . . . " not knowing where she was, accusing her family of things they did not do, running out at night (in the Arctic winter), hearing things other people do not hear, laughing and talking to oneself, tearing off one's clothes, etc. People so afflicted were pointed out to Dr. Murphy without question. The shamans, who went into trances as part of their therapeutic maneuvers, but were otherwise in perfect control of themselves, were never considered crazy by their fellow villagers—this concept had apparently been a result of Ms. Benedict's own preconceptions.

Finally, there is the question of life stresses precipitating psychosis. Although the material just discussed would suggest that this effect is minimal, it not only seems intuitively certain that such an effect exists, but everyone—lay and professional—has seen examples of people "breaking down" because they cannot cope. This is a reasonable point of view, and not at all foreign to medical thinking with respect to ordinary physical illness. However, one caution must be applied to such observations. Patients, and their relatives and friends, often bewildered by what seems to be a sudden onset of physical or mental deterioration, naturally search for a cause. The causes that stand out in their minds are the important landmarks in the patient's life. An unhappy love affair, death of a loved one. Not only may these landmarks be coincidences, but the timing may be stretched to fit the theory.

A laboratory technician in one of the author's laboratories changed from being a superior technician to one who could not concentrate, made serious errors, disappeared for hours during a busy shift, and eventually became incapable of working. He also lost weight, could not sleep and withdrew from most of his social contacts. He went to his general practitioner and told him that the change in his behavior had occurred when he was transferred from a relatively relaxed evening shift to the busy day shift, and the stress was too great for him. The practitioner prescribed a week's vacation and sleeping pills that did no good. On further investigation, including inquiries among the technician's colleagues, it appeared that the behavioral changes had begun to occur *at least* six month's before the shift transfer, but had been rather slow and insidious in developing, and only seemed to require a definite temporal landmark to provide an explanation. The diagnosis was revised to endogenous (not precipitated by outside events) depression, for which the appropriate medication was prescribed with beneficial effect. Within three weeks he was sleeping well, eating better, playing tennis, feeling optimistic, and anticipating going back to work in about another month.

Another example of a changing disease category is childhood autism, an even more distressing condition than schizophrenia, although fortunately with a much lower incidence. The autistic child, apparently normal at birth, very soon shows bizarre mannerisms, such as rocking, head-banging, obsessive behavior, failure to communicate, and failure to learn. It takes a lifetime of effort on the part of the parents to develop in these patients a few habits that will enable them partially to care for themselves. Psychologists and psychiatrists have in the past had a field day blaming parents for bringing on this appalling condition; they blamed domineering mothers and weak fathers, hypocritical pretences of love, and emotional frigidity.

Recent research,[8] however, has shown that of children who are born with signs of intrauterine infection with German measles (signs such as deafness, cataracts, and congenital heart abnormalities), a staggering ten percent or more also become autistic. Incidence of autism in the population as a whole is less than a tenth of a percent! Considering the probability that for every infant known to have been infected with German measles, there are at least three or four who show no detectable signs, and that there are other intrauterine viral infections (such as the jawbreaker, cytomegalic inclusion disease) that are many times more common than German measles, it is quite possible that most or even *all* cases of autism are the result of prenatal viral infection.

Thus it appears that the mental diseases too will simply follow a well-known medical route: from being considered "functional" diseases, for which the symptoms can be observed but the causes and treatments are unknown, to the discovery of treatments that suggest the causes, to the final discovery of the causes and their complete treatments; at this point the disease may be reclassified as anatomic.

It is too much to hope that this final stage will be reached soon. Biological research into mental phenomena is far more difficult than such research into other physical disease and processes. In the first place, animal models are not very useful, since animal parallels to the human psychoses are non-existent or show only weak parallels. Secondly, the usual procedure of examining blood or urine and using the chemical findings in these fluids as a reflection of the processes proceeding in the cells in less effective, because the "blood-brain" barrier guards the secrets of the intracellular chemistry from leaking into the blood. At the very least, spinal fluid (which is much more difficult to obtain) must be used, and even this gives more of a shadow than a reflection of the chemistry that is occurring in the brain.

There also appears to be a peculiar difficulty in determining the specific biochemistry by which genetic changes are transmitted. Of 2500 known genetic traits listed by McCusick in 1975[9] fewer than 200 have an identified biochemical mechanism. Even the original genetic trait, the wrinkling of Mendel's pea, still has an unknown biochemistry! But with the support now being given to biological and biochemical research by the National Institute of Mental Health in the United States, and by similar organizations in many other countries, thoughtful and critical work is now being done everywhere by superior investigators, and we can begin to hope that this final stage of knowledge will not be too long delayed, thus definitively ending the excesses of psychotherapy.

The evidence that all serious mental disease is biologically caused (like diabetes or cancer) is not yet as inherently certain as, for example, is the germ theory of disease, in which the disease can be caused by inocculation of a pure strain of bacteria into a susceptible subject and then transmitted. However, there are few biological facts of any sort that can be demonstrated with this degree of controlled certainty. It is also important to remember that experimentation is impossible in many important fields of science. Astronomers and geologists have for centuries been forced to make deductions from observable phenomena when experiments were impossible, but their results have nonetheless proved remarkably accurate.

In clinical psychiatry, there is readily observable evidence that serious mental disease is biological in origin: to wit, since chemical therapy is by far the most, if not the only, effective treatment for serious mental disease, it would seem reasonable to assume that some chemical flaw in the patient must be in question. Neuroses, which are more likely psychological, do not respond well to biological or chemical treatment.

Let us now examine the mental diseases individually and the therapies currently available. We will begin with the condition known as depression, which is widespread and extremely debilitating. Whether it is a disease or a symptom complex in the sense that cough-fever-and-spitting blood is a symptom complex remains uncertain. What is certain is that through the years there have been a variety of treatments that have shortened or lifted depression, and these treatments have all been biological or chemical.

The first treatment—and one still widely used—was ECT, electroconvulsive therapy, or "shock" treatment. This therapy is based on the observation that depressed patients who had experienced a spontaneous convulsion sometimes enjoyed a remission in their depression. From this grew experimentation in the production of artificial seizures. At first, drugs were used to generate seizures, but these ultimately proved to be dangerous and the results uncertain. The standard method finally arrived at was the introduction of a short duration direct electric current through the brain of the patient by the application of electrodes applied to the scalp. The patient becomes unconscious and convulses; after a course varying from half a dozen to many dozens of treatments, he often improves. In the early use of this therapy, patients frequently fractured their spines, and broke teeth, but concurrent use of muscle relaxants has minimized these side effects. It must be said, however, that most patients are terrified of the experience, and it is uncertain whether there are long-term deleterious side-effects. There is no question that this treatment is often effective in shortening the extremely painful and possibly fatal condition of depression, and perhaps at a time when no other remotely effective treatment modalities were available one could not quibble with the unpleasantness of the technique or its possible side effects.

However, one author feels so strongly that the beneficial effects of ECT have been exaggerated and its harmful effects minimized that he has written a book entitled[10] *Shock Treatment Is Not Good for Your Brain.* He refers to a long series of papers to show that the brains of animals given repeated shock show irreversible damage, which parallels autopsy findings on the few human brains that have been obtainable under similar circumstances, that the heart rate is massively slowed and blood pressure lowered, occasionally sufficiently to kill the patient, and that great changes occur in the endocrine system. These facts would appear to be incontrovertible. He also proposes that permanent memory defects are more common than not, and that in some patients the memory is so permanently disorganized that they are forced to continue their careers at a much lower level. This argument is reminiscent of a lengthy case discussion in the New Yorker[11], which recounted the story of a woman executive who had received a lengthy course of ECT without informed consent for relatively minor reasons and who, although appearing perfectly normal after recovery from her depression, found that she could never again figure out what she was expected to do at her job, eventually lost it, and ended as a volunteer secretary.

Friedberg also asserts that the benefits of ECT are greatly exaggerated. It is his feeling that the procedure is more a punishment than a treatment, and that there would be no loss to therapeutic medicine were it abolished, but rather, a great gain to the patients.

In any event, the chemical antidepressants (vide infra) appear to be supplanting ECT, although some clinicians feel that certain cases of depression that have proved refractory to drug treatment remain amenable to shock therapy as a last resort. The preponderance of modern evidence suggests that when depressives do not respond to medication, either they are not being given the correct dosage, they are not taking it, or, in spite of reasonable dosage, their blood level is low. Blood concentration monitoring may solve the latter problem, and with it, the need for ECT.

At the present time, ECT should be considered a hazardous treatment for which there are good substitutes and should therefore only be used for a specific indication (depression) when alternative therapies (adequately monitored drugs) have failed, only with the consent of the patient or relatives, and probably with two medical opinions.

Other possibilities now exist for the treatment of this condition. The first to appear after ECT was the monoamine oxidase inhibitor (MAOI), one of the current representatives of which is Parnate. Another happy medical accident led to the use of this drug for depression. Some thiry years ago the drug isonicotinic acid hydrazide (INH) had been added to streptomycin to make it a more effective antitubercular drug. It was discovered that tubercular patients who were also depressed had their depression lifted or shortened when they were on these combined drugs, but not when they were on streptomycin alone. Following this, pharmacological and chemical experimentation led to the development of drugs that were not antitubercular, but instead inhibited the monoamine oxidase, as INH had been found to do, and these new drugs proved very helpful in treatment of depression.

Monoamines are a group of chemicals normally secreted by the brain that are involved in transmission of nerve impulses, and include such compounds as serotonin, dopamine, and the relatives of adrenaline. These chemicals are destroyed by an enzyme called monoamine oxidase; the Parnate-like drugs inhibit the action of this destructive enzyme, thereby leading to an increase in the concentration of the monoamines and an increase in their ability to transmit the messages that apparently dispel depression.

There is a clear evolutionary advantage to a brain mechanism that supplies a reasonable optimism to counter the often gloomy prospects of living in a world with a relentlessly hostile environment. Most of us proceed to fill productive roles in life even when the world looks black and hopeless. But for those unfortunates who suffer from endogenous depression, not only do they find it seemingly impossible to cope with the ordinary vicissitudes of life, but they also feel constantly unworthy and unfit. In spite of their own past experiences of happier moments, they can see no end to the present gloom, and suicide seems a most attractive solution, if indeed they still possess the energy to perform the act. Parnate acts by increasing the concentration of those neurotransmitters that apparently are responsible for the ability to maintain a degree of optimism, and the depression lifts within weeks, and sometimes days. Most depressions are self-limited, and a natural remission would usually occur within about six to nine months, even if no medication were used and no change had occurred in the external conditions of the patient, always presuming that suicide had not intervened. Very often, however, periods of depression will recur. This is perhaps an extreme example of a biological rhythm, such as those associated with menstruation, with the daily change in our blood levels of corticosteroids, or with sleep.

The most popular types of antidepressants now in use are the tricyclics, such as Elavil. These chemicals are completely unrelated to the MAOIs, either in chemical structure or physiological behavior. They are much slower-acting, two or three weeks being necessary before any effect is demonstrable in the patient, whereas Parnate may act in days. They are long-acting and need not be taken more than once a day, while Parnate must be given in divided doses. Although the tricyclics are true antidepressants and activate the patient physically as well as emotionally, they have a beneficial sedative effect and, particularly when the daily dose is taken before bedtime, they often supply an uninterrupted night's sleep for the patient who has been waking at three AM for months. Parnate, on the other hand, must not be taken after three or four in the afternoon since it interferes with sleep.

Thus it appears that the two types of antidepressants are complementary, and each should find a use in the treatment of depression. Unfortunately, Parnate has received a bad press and has fallen somewhat into disuse, but it is slowly creeping back into favor again. A number of papers indicated that patients on Parnate could develop serious and acute crises of high blood pressure if they ingested a variety of substances such as red wine, cheese, tinned tuna, or tricyclic antidepressants. Doubt has been cast on some part of these findings by the increasing and effective practice of giving patients both drugs simultaneously. In any event, avoidance of the offending foods removes the hazard, and ought not be considered any more serious a sacrifice for the depressive than avoiding fish or nuts is for the allergic patient.

Before discussing the last useful antidepressant, we must shift to an apparently unrelated and even opposed condition: mania. This condition is almost at the opposite end of the scale from depression. The depressive is hypoactive, sleeping or spending long hours in bed and accomplishing nothing. The manic can literally survive without sleep for days on end and works on innumerable projects at once. The depressive feels completely unworthy and incompetent, while the manic seems constantly bright and energetic. In depression, everything the individual feels or experiences is exaggerated to the point of bject uselessness; the depressive cannot bear the sight or company of others. On the other hand, the manic is overly gregarious. Why then discuss the two in the same paragraph?

Because there is a condition, uncommon but well established, called manic-depressive (or bipolar) psychosis, in which the two states alternate. The alternation may be rapid, and in extremely rare cases, may occur in hours or days. More commonly, the patient may have a manic episode that lasts for some months, return to normal for months, and then repeat the manic episode or have a typical episode of depression. These two conditions, being opposite in behavioral symptoms, would appear to result from opposite distrubances and therefore to require opposite types of therapy. Indeed, the earliest approach to the treatment of mania was more or less opposite to that used for depression, but attempts to sedate, depress, and restrain the overexuberant behavior were more often than not fruitless, since mania is far less tractable than depression. Attempts were also made to use treatment that had been effective with other diseases, for example, ECT, which proved not very useful, and, later, phenothiazines (major tranquilizers), which were of variable effectiveness.

Some thirty years ago, it was found that salts of lithium, a simple inorganic material, were extremely effective in the treatment of acute mania, so that the overactive, overexuberant behavior disappeared—often in a matter of days. Even more important was the observation that the patient was not sedated and that the quality of ideation was restored to normal as rapidly as the overactivity was corrected. Since lithium has virtually no effect on normal people, there was a clear suggestion that it was interfering with or correcting some abnormal pathway that had caused the pathological behavior.

The next step was the attempt to use lithium prophylactically,[12] that is, when the patient is well, in the hopes of preventing recurrences. Not only was the salt found to be useful in this way, but it was discovered that the depressive episodes often following the manic phase were aborted, delayed, or rendered less serious and deep. From this evidence the impression arose that lithium was a specific remedy for manic-depressive disease, as therapy for acute mania, and as a prophylaxis in the long term for both the manic and depressive episodes of bipolar manic-depressive disease. Many psychiatrists still believe that this is its only use.

Although it is gratifying to have available a drug that is so effective in treating a mental disorder, it would not be too important, except in its theoretical implications, if this was all it was good for because true manic-depressive illness is relatively rare, even among the population of mental patients. The real significance of lithium seems to be that it is of prophylactic value in some patients who suffer unipolar depression,[13] that is, recurrent depressive episodes with no suggestion of mania at any time. It also appears to be somewhat effective in controlling the symptoms of mania not uncommonly associated with schizophrenia (so-called "schizoaffective variety"), even when it is not connected with manic-depressive illness.[14] It is for these reasons that lithium is looked upon with such hope, not only by progressive medical practitioners, but by a great army of sufferers who have read of its broad spectrum of therapeutic uses in the lay press. The side effects and cautions required in the use of this drug have already been discussed.

We now come to the most serious and destructive disease or group of diseases of the mind or brain: the schizophrenias. At least two percent of the entire human race suffers from this condition, and fifty percent of all mental hospital beds are occupied by schizophrenics. The disease is usually chronic and, until a few years ago, it usually meant life-long incarceration in a mental hospital.

The picture is now reasonably different, although the disease continues to manifest in much the same way, and with much the same prevalence. Symptoms of the untreated disease still include hallucinations, imperfect perception and understanding of reality, fearful nightmares, paranoia, and progressive incapacity to work, enjoy life, and to form stable relationships. But the difference in the last thirty years has been that the group of drugs called the phenothiazines have been used effectively with these patients.

The history of the development of the phenothiazines begins with antihistamines, the drugs that are used to control symptoms of hayfever and other allergic phenomena. When it was found that one of the unpleasant side effects of many antihistamines was a tendency to cause drowsiness, medical researchers utilized it to control the bizarre behavior of some schizophrenics. Some slight successes led the researchers to make chemical modifications of the drug, thereby creating a new class of drugs: the ataractics, major tranquilizers, or antipsychotic drugs. The phenothiazines, such as chlorpromazine, Stelazine, and Mellaril, fall into this category. These drugs cannot restore the pre-morbid personality, because they do not cure, they only control; but they make it possible for seventy to eighty percent of patients using them to function at least part of the time outside an institution. They are infinitely more important in restoring the patient to such a state than any amount of psychotherapy, milieu, conditioning, or any other psychological maneuvering. In most cases where they have proved ineffective, the drugs are found to have been prescribed in inadequate amounts, or the patient has not been taking the drugs as prescribed.

It is very difficult for the schizophrenic to maintain a lifelong regimen of psychotropic drugs. In the first place, these drugs all have unpleasant side effects; frequently they cause a Parkinson-like syndrome of stiffness, tremor, and rigidity. In many patients these symptoms need to be controlled by other drugs, which also have side effects. Luckily, some of these symptoms disappear with prolonged use. Almost all the drugs mentioned cause dryness of the nose and mouth, plus slight impairment of the vision. Some of them cause the blood pressure to fall when the patient stands up. Some cause impotence and failure to ejaculate.

These unpleasant side effects are, admittedly, small prices to pay for being able to function outside an institution, but the world conspires against faithful adherence to the prescription. All patients have friends who assure them that they can pull themselves up by their bootstraps and not use drugs as a crutch. And unfortunately the physician and the social worker who are trying to help the patient may be ambivalent in their feelings about the medication and may suggest that some type of mental exertion can take its place. The "revolving door" effect in which the hospitalized patient is discharged much improved, only to reappear months later in desperate condition is often the consequence of the patient being taken off needed drugs by some well-meaning team in the community health program that has been charged with his or her welfare.

Unhappily, it seems that in our social order, the daily self-administration of pills to maintain sanity serves as a constant reproach to patients. They are made to feel that they ought to be able to keep their own "minds" in line without taking pills. No one, of course, suggests that people must keep their own diseased hearts, livers, kidneys, or gall bladders in line without pills.

The final difficulty facing the patient on medication is the efficacy of the drugs. Once the drugs have made patients feel better, they question whether they were ever ill at all, quit taking their medication, and slide insidiously into a state of ill health and impaired judgment that prevents them from returning to their medication. Patients with hypothyroidism, pernicious anemia, and even diabetes go through this same cycle of treatment, apparent cure, withdrawal of medication, and re-hospitalization.

As with lithium, along with the annoying but harmless side effects comes a serious and potentially irreversible one—*tardive dyskinesia.* This rare but apparently increasingly found side effect, which often manifests itself some considerable time after the drug is discontinued, and which particularly afflicts patients over the age of 50, causes involuntary movements not dissimilar to those seen in chorea (St. Vitus' dance). Even more distressing than these movements of the limbs are the peculiar involuntary facial grimaces so often found; these generally make the patient's social adjustment even more difficult than it already is.

It is not yet certain how many cases of tardive dyskinesia are reversible, or whether reported treatments to correct it are effective. Fortunately, in comparison with what we presently know about lithium, the incidence of tardive dyskinesia seems to be directly correlated with the total amount of drug taken and with continuous use of the drug. It is for this reason that some of the most careful clinics, such as the Clarke Institute Clinic described elsewhere, institute routine drug holidays and attempt always to use the smallest dose that will rehabilitate the patient, even if it does not remove all symptoms.

The discussion of the biogenic theory and chemical treatment of mental disease would be incomplete without mentioning one of the special approaches in this category: the megavitamin or orthomolecular school. This group of physicians and scientists believe that mental illness, as well as many other types of physical illness, are caused by an abnormal metabolism of normal components in the diet that leads to an imperfect internal chemical environment resulting in disease. For example, it is believed by some orthomolecular psychiatrists that schizophrenics need to ingest dozens or hundreds of times the usual amount of niacin (vitamin B_3) to obtain the usual protective effects. Indeed, the principal in one of the cases reported in this book is now well and attending graduate school on a regimen of carefully controlled diet and high vitamin B_6 dosage, *without* psychotropic drugs.

Although the tenets of the orthomolecular school are not widely accepted by the medical profession, they have been of incalculable benefit to many sufferers from mental illness and their relatives. This school, associated with the name of Abram Hoffer,[15] and later Linus Pauling,[16] in arguing for their ideas of therapy, have produced the most cogent arguments available on the biological nature of mental disease, thereby lifting the load of guilt that had often been deposited by Freudian and other psychologically inclined therapists on the shoulders of patients and relatives, people who were already carrying the almost intolerable burden of one of the most chronic and heartbreaking diseases known. This destruction of false guilts will never be forgotten by the thousands who have read their works, whether or not they have benefited from or even tried orthomolecular treatment.

Most of the medications that have been discussed here are not as well-known to the general public as Valium and Librium, which are representatives of a group of drugs known as the benzodiazepines. These drugs have taken the place of barbiturates as the most commonly used psychoactive drugs, and tens of millions of North Americans with many different complaints take them as anti-anxiety agents.

The benzodiazepines are of little or no use in the treatment of psychoses, the serious mental disorders with which we are most concerned, and they are seldom knowingly prescribed for such conditions. However, anxiety may be a symptom of a serious underlying disorder such as depression. If such an anxiety is treated with a benzodiazepine, it not only fails to help, but may actually increase the depression, since benzodiazepines, like barbiturates, are depressing drugs. Furthermore, the patient soon develops a tolerance to these medications and requires constant increases in the dosage. (This is also true of barbiturates and narcotics, but not of the antipsychotics and antidepressants.) Psychological dependency often develops as well. Then the progress of the illness develops as follows: a depressed patient with anxiety symptoms is put on the benzodiazepines, and then becomes more deeply depressed although there is initial relief from anxiety. A tolerance to the drug is developed, the dosage must be increased, the depression deepens, and suffering from insomnia necessitates supplementation with sleeping pills, which further aggravates the depression. If the same patient is put on antidepressants, most of the time the depression and anxiety will lessen, sleep will be better, and faster recovery will ensue.

Many physicians still prescribe benzodiazepines rather than tricyclic antidepressants because they believe the former are very safe and relatively ineffective in suicide attempts. Indeed the amount of Librium or Valium required to kill someone is very large, but more and more hospital admissions are now occurring because of overdoses of these medications. Additionally, Librium and Valium are increasingly being implicated in automobile accidents. Many physicians are asking themselves whether ineffectiveness is a reasonable price to pay for low toxicity.

These then are the basic medical facts of psychiatry. That they are ignored by many practitioners of this specialty is obvious from the case studies we are here reporting.

6

Facing Reality

> There are more things in Heaven and Earth, Horatio, than are dreamt of in your philosophy.
>
> —Shakespeare

Paula Green is now twenty-eight years old; she is the second child in a family of four. She first became depressed at the age of eighteen, but determinedly coped with it for a few years without medical help. In this interview Paula speaks of the most difficult years of her illness.

Question: Paula, you've seen a number of psychiatrists in your search for health. Would you describe the type of treatment you've received?
Paula: Of course. I guess I should talk about Dr. Kane first because I went to him for over five years. There are many things about him that I admire and respect, and there were times when he really gave me excellent care on an emotional level. But he failed in the management of my illness and he just ignored my physical complaints.
Question: What kind of treatment did Dr. Kane use?
Paula: Well, mostly group therapy, but Dr. Kane really has an eclectic approach to therapy. You could almost say he changed his approach abruptly from year to year.
Question: What did you discuss in group therapy?
Paula: Well, I didn't have any major life problems to

discuss so I had to invent some to stay there—I was in a hospital at the time. But the full program they tried to put me on would have been hard to take. They used to instigate people to attack one another, you understand, but I was too depressed and so I never really became involved. I didn't have any self-esteem left by that time. So that winter Dr. Kane decided to try Glasser's Reality Therapy[1] on me. I'd been so deeply depressed for so many months that he thought this might lift me out of it. His other approaches had been totally ineffectual, although they had been on the whole kind and quite humane. But Reality Therapy, as he applied it to me, wasn't either kind or humane after it passed that initial phase.

Question: Can you describe the initial phase?

Paula: Oh, the first phase involved forming a very intense personal relationship between doctor and patient, and in order to form it, the doctor has to be totally accepting of the patient. In my case, this was great, since I was suffering from depression and I had a real need for complete, unconditional acceptance. However, after Dr. Kane had told me that he was "the most important person" in my life and had convinced me through our close relationship that I couldn't get along with him, his treatment became really harsh and cruel. He told me that I was childish and immature and that he was going to "grow me up" no matter how much I resisted. This really upset me as I knew that I was no more immature than other people my own age. What he was calling immaturity and childishness were just symptoms of my illness. Then he began to imply that I was irresponsible. Now I'd always considered myself to be a fairly responsible person so this really disturbed me. But I know now that in Reality Therapy anyone who is unable to fulfill the two essential needs—to love and to be loved, and to feel worthwhile to oneself and to others—is considered irresponsible. Glasser says that people are not irresponsible because they are ill, but rather, that they are ill because they are irresponsible. The patient's irresponsibility lies in being unable to fulfill these two needs. But *anyone* who is experiencing a depression will feel unloved and worthless, and surely it doesn't follow that they are irresponsible because they feel this way! But because I felt this way, I wasn't considered ill by Dr. Kane, simply irresponsible, and this just increased the load of guilt and self-recrimination I was already carrying around. Finally, this change in Dr. Kane's behavior toward me—from accepting me as I was to ignoring my illness and laying expectations on me that I couldn't meet because I was really ill—drove me to the edge of suicide. That summer, I soaked my clothes with gasoline and was going to set myself on fire because I was convinced that this was the right and just punishment for a person who behaved badly and irresponsibly. And before that, I hadn't attempted suicide for over eight months, although I'd been just as depressed during that time as I was that summer. I'm sure my attempt to kill myself came from the fact that there'd been no improvement in my condition for over a year—plus the pressure of Reality Therapy. Even Glasser himself admits it can be dangerous!

Question: Before we proceed with the Reality Therapy, I would like to return to a statement you just made: "...[expectations] I couldn't meet because I was really ill." Could you describe this illness in more detail?

Paula: Well, ever since my last year in high school I had been steadily going down hill. I had absolutely no energy. I went to bed as soon as I got home from school. My school work deteriorated. I felt worthless and bad. It became more and more difficult for me to hold down a job. And I didn't have any intervals in which this illness lifted, nor did any treatment help me.

Question: Did Dr. Kane give you any medication during this period?

Paula: At various times he had me on imipramine or Parnate. None of it seemed to help.

This description of unremitting physical fatigue, and perhaps weakness (weakness being an objective sign rather than simply a feeling, as fatigue is), along with the psychic manifestations of depression, suggest strongly that Paula was indeed suffering from a true physical illness. As will be seen in the sequel, she may well be afflicted with a biochemical abnormality characterizable even with our present knowledge if her doctors had cared to investigate.

Dr.Kane's attempt to bully a person almost certainly burdened with a severe physical illness into pulling herself up by her own bootstraps suggests a number of the more extreme cases collected by Dr. Irving Cooper in his book,[2] *The Victim is Always the Same.* Dr. Cooper presents several cases of a rare disease called Dystonia Musculorum Deformans (DMD), in which a deterioration of nerve cells in the brain results in a locking of the limbs of the victim into grotesque and functionless attitudes, thereby making normal activity impossible. In every case discussed by Dr. Cooper, the patients were referred quickly to psychoanalytically inclined physicians who diagnosed them as hysterics, psychosomatics, or with other psychological labels, and then proceeded to the most inhumane kind of mistreatment imaginable.

Susan was a typical case. After a long course of otherwise unsuccessful therapy, she was eventually forced to crawl on the ice to her school bus one morning in the belief that this application of "Reality" would cause her to desist from what the psychotherapist considered to be her manipulative and spurious paralysis. The family naturally argued the pros and cons of this kind of treatment, and their quarrels ultimately culminated in a physical attack on the mother by the father. Eventually Susan arrived at Dr. Cooper's office, where she was correctly diagnosed as suffering from DMD, treated by his method of cryosurgery (freezing some of the brain cells), and subsequently made a reasonable recovery.

The almost willful persistence of the psychologically oriented doctors in their grossly inaccurate diagnoses led Sir Peter Medawar, in his review of Dr. Cooper's book[2a] to say, "the opinion is gaining ground that doctrinaire psychoanalysis [one could add many of the newer-fangled psychotherapies that are discussed in this book] is the most stupendous intellectual confidence trick of the 20th century: and a terminal product as well—something akin to a dinosaur or a zeppelin in the history of ideas, a vast structure of radically unsound design and with no posterity."

> *Question:* You've obviously done considerable reading on Reality Therapy technique.
> *Paula:* Yes, I did. I had to understand what had happened to me.
> *Question:* Did you stay with Dr. Kane after your suicide attempt?
> *Paula:* Yes. Dr. Kane had been pressuring me to make plans and get on with my life according to the principles of Reality Therapy. So in September, after not working for over a year, I got a job in a lab. I was certain that this would please him, but when I phoned and told him, he didn't show any interest at all. I was devastated! It seemed like there was nothing I could do to please him. And I wanted desperately to do exactly that. From my reading I now understand that he didn't act pleased because Glasser's Reality Therapy holds as a basic tenet that people feel worthless because they have too low expectations for themselves. So if patients are capable of more than what they are doing according to the therapist's opinion, they should not receive praise, but instead be directed towards those things that will better allow them to fulfill their potential. The only action I could take to be deserving of Dr. Kane's praise was go back to university and take graduate studies. So, trying to please him, even though I was barely hanging together, I applied for two correspondence courses, but was too sick to do the courses and just threw away several hundred dollars. Therapy can be a mighty expensive proposition even when it's mostly being paid for by social or health insurance of some sort! The problem was that I suffered from the misguided notion that if I could please Dr. Kane,

I would be making progress and I'd eventually get better. Some hope! I never got well under *any* therapy Dr. Kane applied to me and I grew steadily *worse* under Reality Therapy.

Question: You left Dr. Kane eventually?

Paula: Yes, after about five years—we had quite an argument! He told me that he "didn't want to be stuck with me for the rest of his life!" I felt that if that was the way he felt about me I was certainly not going to impose my unpleasant personality on him. And I decided that *never* under any circumstances would I allow another psychiatrist to treat me. I made up my mind to stay away from them and their hospitals no matter how much I suffered!

I was totally disillusioned by a medical profession that kept telling me that I was a fine healthy girl when I wasn't even able to get out of bed, or take a bath, or do anything without my insides shaking so much that other people could feel them. Then my mother begged me to try the orthomolecular approach and I agreed in order to please her because I felt I would soon be dead anyhow.

You know, within twenty-four hours of being placed on huge doses of pyridoxine (Vitamin B_6) my depression lifted for the first time. Finally, there's no doubt at all in my mind that I was really ill—not just irresponsible! And I know that Dr. Kane didn't have the right to apply Reality Therapy to me, because even Glasser says that Reality Therapy shouldn't be used until all organic causes have been ruled out.

Question: Does Dr. Kane still practice this technique?

Paula: Oh yes. He uses it at City Hospital and has treated over 600 patients in group therapy there. That technique has no scientific basis or validity. It's humanly unsound, and as far as I know, he doesn't follow up patients. Sometime you should have a look at the psychiatric short- and long-stay units there during visiting hours and read the signs that they have posted about the treatment approach. I don't believe that Dr. Kane would object.

> He's extremely proud of what he's doing there. Possibly he'd even be willing to talk about it with you because he's willingly discussed it with me since then. There might be some hope of encouraging him to adopt the orthomolecular approach because he's tried everything else. Of course, he's afraid of social disapproval.

Paula's hope that Dr. Kane might adopt the orthomolecular approach stemmed from one of her early contacts with him when he told her that she was suffering from a biochemical imbalance, but he didn't know what it was. Like many psychiatrists he vacillated between belief in the biological versus the psychological nature of mental illness, but acted almost entirely on the psychological theory.

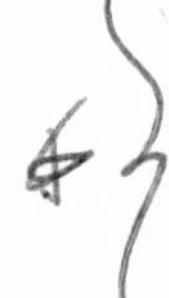

As part of this psychological treatment, Dr. Kane's rejection of Paula was potentially the most dangerous maneuver. Given her history of suicide attempts, including her attempt at self-immolation, and the fact that he had almost convinced her that her failure to get well was her own fault, it is only by great fortune that she did not kill herself.

This horrifying episode inevitably raises the distressing question of the fate of other patients who are rejected by their psychiatrists. When such strong bonds are created between patients and doctors, do patients have the will to continue living when they are abandoned? What is the suicide rate among patients who are treated as Paula was?

We would like to be able to answer this question. And so would Dr. Alan A. Stone of Harvard Medical School and Harvard Law School. "Put starkly," he asks,[3] "can psychotherapy precipitate or contribute to a suicide? A review of the *Psychological Abstracts* over the past ten years reveals hundreds of scientific articles on suicide, but not one deals specifically with this question . . . I have presented clinical case material which I think demonstrates that psychotherapy can precipitate suicide or serious suicide attempts." Dr. Stone feels that these suicides or suicide attempts are contributed to by the psychiatrist's establishment of a symbiotic relationship with the patient from which he finally backs away in fear or dismay.

The question whether psychotherapy represents "benign or malignant intervention" is also raised in several other papers and books. Tennov's *Psychotherapy, the Hazardous Cure*[4] deals at length with the question. A study from Vanderbilt University called[5] *Contemporary Views of Negative Effects in Psychotherapy* queries many leading psychiatrists and concludes that "it is clear that negative effects of psychotherapy are overwhelmingly regarded by experts in the field as a significant problem requiring the attention and concern of practitioners and researchers alike." They call attention to the instigation of "ill-fated attempts by the patient to overreach his capabilities, and, as a result of any or all of these specific negative effects, disillusionment with the therapist or with therapy in general," exactly as Paula complained.

An interesting side issue is the rather consistent use by the critics of psychotherapy of the word "negative" to describe harmful effects. In all other branches of medicine, the standard term used in indexing such effects is "adverse." The use of the ambiguous and colorless term "negative" to replace it almost suggests that the critics cannot bring themselves to feel that psychotherapy may sometimes be as harmful as, for example, medication or surgery. However, the word "deleterious" effects of psychotherapy is beginning to appear more frequently in the literature and in lectures.

In spite of the uneasiness expressed by these authorities, we have not been able to find a statistical study aimed at answering the questions. Indeed, under present conditions, the statistical material is not available. This lack has led a Canadian body, the Committee of Concern for Mental Patients, to write a letter to Medical Examiners and Coroners suggesting that the following questions should be asked in the investigation of all suicides:

1. Was the deceased under the care of a physician/psychiatrist?
2. What was the nature of the treatment? Was confrontation used?
3. Were they on medication(s) and if so, what were they and in what dosage were they used. If not, why not?

When the answers to such questions become part of vital statistics, it will be possible to begin to do research on the effect of psychotherapy and medication on suicide, possibly leading to more significant attempts at prevention than are now available.

Although there seems to have been little research on the questions raised here, there is no paucity of literature on the psychological effects of patients' suicide on their therapists. Merton J. Kahne, research psychiatrist at MIT, describes the reaction of psychiatrists whose patients have committed suicide.[6] "The suicide is almost always taken by the therapist as a direct act of spite against him . . . Many therapists refer to the event as being 'fired'." Dr. Donald W. Light describes a psychiatrist who said,[7] "She fought me all the way, and I guess she finally made her point."

Contributing to the difficulty of obtaining any reasonable analysis of the problem is the denial mechanism with which it is approached by many therapists. Dr. Light, in the study quoted above, remarks, "One psychiatrist had said of a patient just prior to her suicide attempt that she was 'not suicidal.' Another said the same thing of a patient who had just killed himself." Dr. Ralph H. Henn in a study of suicides occurring during the psychiatric residency[8] discusses 23 suicides under 20 residents. "Of these 20 residents, 19 were totally unaware of the suicides."

I followed through on Paula's suggestion that I visit Dr. Kane's hospital unit. I asked him whether patients could be excused from group therapy sessions if they felt too fragile or if their personalities were too private. He replied that they might take one or possibly two days leave, but after that they'd have to go to a hotel if they needed a rest. Dr. Kane was not going to waste taxpayer's money on patients who refused to attend group therapy.

Dr. Kane in his unvalidated fixation on encounter group methods was unable to realize that the personalities of many patients lead them to find the excessive sharing of intimacies quite repugnant. And this personality is not peculiar to patients. Somerset Maugham says of himself,[9] "I have no desire to lay bare my heart and I put limits to intimacy . . . . I am content to maintain my privacy." For such patients, it would be far more beneficial were they to enter some quiet rest home, or, as Alan Watts once said, "some patients need an Ashram—a place to repair, a place to rest."

We now return to the fascinating question of what was actually responsible for Paula's near-miraculous recovery. On re-reading her interview, we gathered that she felt the orthomolecular treatment had reversed the course of her long-standing disease in a matter of days. This seemed so incredible upon reflection that we made a trip to the university town in which she now lives to discover whether we or she had misinterpreted the events of her illness and subsequent return to health. Paula very kindly consented to be questioned in great detail, almost as a witness in a courtroom. The following facts were elicited.

First, her illness was progressive and unremitting for about seven years. She had struggled through university, she knew not how. She became progressively less able to do her school work or engage in gainful employment. After her graduation and summer rest, she went to another city and registered in a graduate school, where she accomplished nothing for the first semester. Returning home for Christmas, she went promptly to bed and stayed there for some months. Attempts to work failed. She then attempted graduate work in Business Administration during the following September, at which she lasted a week. At this point, she gave up. "I wasn't even suicidal any more because I was convinced I was going to die, so what was the use of making the effort."

Paula, who had by this time given up reading as well as all other pursuits, was not looking for a solution. It was her mother who discovered the orthomolecular literature and decided that Paula needed pyridoxine. She persuaded Paula to take the staggering dose of 3000 mg daily (the U.S. National Research Council Recommended Daily Allowance is 2 mg). After three days Paula was so improved that she remembers to this day, "I never realized people could feel like that." Since then she has become completely normal, both physically and mentally. She continues to take large doses (1000 mg) of pyridoxine with other vitamins and minerals. She has completed two additional years of University science with sufficiently high marks to be admitted to graduate school, where she will study biochemistry. She has had only one relapse in three years. This lasted three days and was terminated by the addition of folic acid to her regimen.

It seems difficult to attribute her recovery to some other factor than does Paula herself. Unremitting progressive depression with bizarre behavior such as she describes simply does not come to an end spontaneously in three or four days. Even if one could believe that pyridoxine had such a powerful placebo effect, Paula would be an unlikely candidate to experience that effect because she was simply taking the vitamin to please her mother, and not because she had any belief in it.

Although there is as yet no well-authenticated case in the literature of a psychosis being cured by large doses of pyridoxine, there is one in which folic acid plays such a role.[10] The patient at age twelve developed a marked schizophrenic reaction, with delusions, hallucinations, and catatonia. It was ultimately found that she had a cellular defect in her folic acid metabolic pathway, and large doses of folic acid corrected the schizophrenia. The disease could then be turned on and off by withholding and administering this vitamin. Since the girl was mentally subnormal and did not understand what was being done to her, there was no possibility of a placebo effect governing her reactions.

Turning again to Paula, and assuming that the vitamins indeed cured her, what are we to think? Is she a rare case of pyridoxine dependency, just as there are rare infants whose convulsions can be cured by high doses of pyridoxine? Or would many mental patients benefit by this treatment? Many enzymes that produce the important brain transmitters whose lack are generally considered to contribute to mental disorder have pyridoxal phosphate as a coenzyme. If there were some difficulty in securing an adequate concentration of pyridoxal phosphate in an individual's brain, such a person would likely suffer a mental disorder and it seems possible that massive doses of pyridoxine might correct the disorder.

In our view, it might well prove an important step in the history of brain research if Paula were to submit herself to experiments in which pyridoxine was alternately withdrawn and restored while her mental and biochemical state was closely monitored. Although she is a scientific person who would like to see this experiment done, she is naturally quite reluctant, at this stage in her career, to attempt to provoke a return to the state from which she suffered for so many years, and, indeed, it is a serious ethical question for the scientists who would advocate and supervise such a test whether they have the right to ask such a sacrifice of her, or indeed anyone.

7

Treatment by Assault

When Ray and Jocelyn Ans were married, she was a well-known actress, and he was a successful laboratory physician. It was a second marriage for both of them, and though each of them had been childless in their first marriage, they now had two children.

After ten years of fairly harmonious marriage, Jocelyn began to withdraw from her family and friends. She took to drinking, and often refused to leave her bed for days at a time. She began talking of suicide, and even went so far as to buy various poisons while she decided which one was suitable. At other times she became a wild woman and attacked her husband verbally, and on one occasion she even attacked him physically. Her behavior is reminiscent of Virginia Woolf's, of whom Harold Nicholson once said, "When Virginia was mad, she was totally mad; she bit and scratched, and heard the birds talking Greek in the garden."

Ray's interview continues the story.

> *Ray:* About the time that happened (the physical attack), I attended a lecture by a well-known psychiatrist, Dr. Harkness it was, and he really impressed me as a man who would have some solutions for us. So I went to see him and I told him about Joss. Well, he listened and then he said that she was just acting up and misbehaving, that she should be treated like a naughty child. He advised me to slap her when she next behaved that way, and to lock her out of the house. This really went against the grain with

me! I'd never done anything like that—I'd never even *thought* of doing it. But this was professional advice from a university-based physician who was an acknowledged expert. So on the *next* occasion when Joss misbehaved, I picked her up and put her outside the back door. She resisted, of course, and tried to hold onto objects as we went along, but I shut the back door and locked her out. The result of all this was that she screamed so loud and long—and being an actress she's got a pretty penetrating voice—that eventually I thought: "Well, this is a pretty stupid procedure!" and I let her in.

Question: Did this psychiatrist make any suggestions concerning the cause of Jocelyn's problems or inquire about the nature of your own relationship with her?

Ray: It's difficult for me to recall, because as time went on I think we were involved with at least three, or perhaps four, different psychiatrists, so I can't be absolutely sure. I believe Dr. Harkness said he would not suggest a divorce at that time. Of course, we only saw him over a short period—but it is possible he may have suggested separation—I'm not sure about that.

Question: What happened to Jocelyn as a result of this episode?

Ray: Well, I don't know whether this was a direct result, but she retreated to her bed again a little later and became completely unresponsive. Finally she had to be admitted to the university teaching hospital for psychotherapy. I remember that she was required to recall all the events since her birth. When she came out of hospital she was somewhat calmer and seemed able to function more normally, but after a while the wildness and talk of suicide started all over again. Then one night when I was away—I'd just come to the end of my tolerance I guess—she actually wound up in our district hospital emergency ward from a drug overdose. It was traumatic at the time, but it was there that we started with another psychiatrist, who for the first time attempted to evaluate her biochemistry, and that was the beginning of her recovery.

Question: Was she put on medication at that time? What about supportive therapy for her?

Ray: Well actually yes, Joss got supportive therapy from the doctor—he was a general practitioner—who admitted her at the time and he believed in such therapeutic approaches as hypnosis and was very good with her, eventually bringing in a psychiatrist to help. But as far as I'm concerned, the supportive therapy I myself provided went back much further than that—although it wasn't until she became so much improved from her new medication that supportive therapy was going to make much headway with her. Incidentally, she was put on the antipsychotic Stelazine then, and previously she'd been denied Stelazine because of her low white blood count. The doctor discovered that her white blood count went up and down independently of the Stelazine, which therefore couldn't have caused the low count. In fact her counts have decreased only marginally since she's been on it.

All that time she had been denied the benefits of Stelazine because they hadn't bothered to investigate. In point of fact, of course, Jocelyn really had never been given a proper physical examination or laboratory investigation until she entered our own hospital where she was observed for two or three weeks without medication but with daily blood tests; ultimately they put her on both thyroid and Stelazine.

It seems to me that under the present system, psychiatrists practice too frequently like special psychologists; they evidently don't always treat patients as the physicians they are. In theory you must first be a doctor before entering psychiatric training so that you know all about the pathology and the physical aspects of mental disease. You see, until Joss was admitted to a general hospital under the care of a general practitioner she was not really examined physically nor was she properly investigated pathologically. If psychiatrists limit themselves to what they call psychotherapy, then why do they need to be doctors at all?

Ray's indignation at the repeated neglect of ordinary medical principles in the approach to Jocelyn's illness is amply justified by a copious literature demonstrating that depending on the study, between 5 and 43% of the psychiatric complaints that brought patients to a hospital or clinic were caused by diagnosable physical illnesses. A considerable portion of the remaining patients suffered exacerbations of their mental illness because of concomitant physical complaints, and many others had unrelated physical illnesses.

These startling figures have been produced because some psychiatric clinics make a practice of not admitting patients unless they receive a complete and competent physical examination together with a thorough laboratory investigation and X-rays and other special procedures when indicated. Dr. E. K. Koranyi of the department of psychiatry at Ottawa University reports on 1090 psychiatric clinic patients who were examined in this way.[1] He found that 43% suffered from one or more physical illnesses and that about half these illnesses had not been diagnosed by the referring source. Psychiatrists and psychiatric institutes missed 48% of the medical diagnoses, whereas other referring physicians did slightly better, missing only 32%. A startling 69% of the physical illnesses "contributed considerably to the psychiatric state of the patients." Among the physically ill, 18% of the mental illnesses resulted exclusively from the underlying physical illness, about 9% of the total patients. The mental diagnoses ran the whole gamut of psychoses and neuroses, and the causative or aggravating physical illnesses encompassed infections, tumors, endocrine diseases, including many instances of diabetes mellitus, hypoglycemia, and thyroid disease, hypertensive heart disease, diseases of the urinary tract, systemic lupus erythematosis, and so on. In another article entitled[2] *Physical Illness Presenting as Psychiatric Disease,* R. C. Hall and colleagues produced remarkably similar figures showing that among 658 consecutive psychiatric clinic patients who received careful medical and biochemical evaluation, 9.1% had causative medical disorders. Again, the whole spectrum of physical disease is implicated, but the variety of mental diseases is somewhat smaller, possibly because of the type of patient treated at Hall's institution. His group reviewed the literature, and found their experience to be quite typical, and concluded with a plea for renewed attention to the careful medical evaluation of psychiatric patients.

A dramatic case history was published by Cerkez and Ferguson.[3] A traveling salesman in his thirties began showing signs of agitated depression that often became worse on his trips away from home. He finally required admission to a mental hospital, where he became violent. He was treated with electroconvulsive shock and discharged "improved." However, the "improvement" did not last and he was again admitted on several other occasions. On one of these occasions, he reached the emergency department of the London, Ontario General Hospital where Dr. Ferguson examined him and suspected that he might be suffering from hypoglycemia. A glucose tolerance test showed blood sugars quite low enough to account for his symptoms. The shape of the glucose tolerance curve also showed that the patient was an early diabetic. Treatment for his diabetes cured the symptoms.

A fascinating sequel to this story occurred when the authors of this book wrote to Dr. Ferguson eight years later to ask whether the patient had remained well or whether he had had coexisting mental and physical disease. The reply was an excited phone call to reassure us that the patient was well and active in business and had experienced no relapses, but—of almost greater interest—that his brother had been admitted to emergency that day with identical symptoms and equally low blood sugar!

As we have seen, Ray was advised by a psychiatrist to assault his wife physically, but was too civilized to follow this advice. That his psychiatrist is not the only one who believes in using physical assault as an integral component of psychotherapy is shown by the experience of Kit, in a Day Care Center whose staff were ardently devoted to far-out therapies.

Kit, who is a social worker, thirty five, and mother of three, made an attempt at suicide. After she was discharged from hospital, she was referred to the Day Care Center for follow-up therapy, which she initially felt had benefited her. "Everybody liked me; I felt more self-worth and camaraderie."

One morning, when Kit arrived at the Day Care Center, the psychiatrist in charge brought out the mat and directed Kit to lie down on it. He then asked the patients with whom she had been working most closely to hold her down, knelt over her, and "proceeded to beat me up. He slapped my face until my nose bled, punched me in the ribs until I was black and blue. I thought he had broken a rib. I rushed away home, sobbing and crying. And I thought they were all my friends."

The pathethic conclusion of this unbelievable incident of assault, in which bodily and psychic injury was inflicted by a man who had sworn the Hippocratic oath to do the patient no harm, is that Kit, who had recovered almost completely from her suicidal depression, suffered another psychotic attack and once again had to be committed to hospital for treatment.

To return to Ray, at the end of the interview, he spoke of the general practitioner's ability to cope with the varied aspects of each patient's illness. Any physician, he said, knows that the physical rehabilitation of the patient after illness greatly depends on psychological factors; a patient won't get well without the necessary will. He then told a story that suggests that some psychiatrists use this kind of knowledge improperly:

> At one time a young woman was on a work adjustment program in our lab. She had just come from a psychiatric ward and was doing exceptionally well, mixing with the other women, when one day she retreated into silence, abandoning her formerly friendly social traits. Her associates asked her what was wrong. She told them that

> the psychiatrist had told her that she was becoming too dependent on them, which I had felt was the very thing that was helping her—mixing with them—and she then went on to say that he'd told her that she would never be well and would always need him! But thank goodness, she eventually got well, and in retrospect, it doesn't appear at all that she *does* need him!

On the other hand, some psychiatrists write about an exemplary technique for managing schizophrenics—the most difficult group of mental patients. Dr. Mary Seeman[4] describes the results of a three year study at the Clarke Institute of Psychiatry outpatient clinic in Toronto designed to discover optimal methods of treating schizophrenics. They conclude that the ability of their patients to survive in the community is seriously affected because they have usually become ill in adolescence, before they have developed work and interpersonal skills; because their lives have been interrupted by several stays in hospital; and because they are usually unemployed, indigent, malnourished, and isolated. Treatment is therefore directed toward keeping the patient on optimum medication, enlisting help from staff, family, and friends. Missed appointments are followed up and the patient is cajoled into attending clinic. Group sessions are flexible, nonconfrontative, supportive, and well attended. Doctors are accessible at all times. Patients are carefully observed for the side effects of medications, and these are kept at the lowest dose that effectively relieves most of the symptoms. In an attempt to minimize late side effects, patients are given drug holidays under even closer observation than usual, with medication reinstituted as soon as symptoms recur. The general health of the patient is looked after as is their lodging and nutrition.

It would be difficult to think of any major improvements

for such a humane and medically effective program. Possibly more effort could be directed to providing employment, but such a course might require resources that the Clarke Institute does not possess.

A slightly different approach is used by Ronald R. Fieve at the New York State Psychiatric Institute. In an article,[5] *The Lithium Clinic: A New Model for the Delivery of Psychiatric Services*, Fieve, a pioneer in the use of lithium, describes fifteen years of experience in his clinic. Whereas the Clarke Institute clinic is dealing with outpatient schizophrenics, Fieve treats patients with affective disorders (depression, manic–depressive disease, etc.). He finds that such patients outnumber schizophrenics by at least a factor of three and possibly a factor of ten. Careful attention is paid to diagnosis (thus correcting one of the failings of American psychiatry) and the mainstay of treatment is then lithium, although other drugs are used as necessary. Patients are seen regularly at monthly intervals for clinical evaluation, lithium monitoring, and behavior and mood ratings. A physician is called only if some problem arises. The entire group is seen in one two-hour period a month. Although "the staff makes little attempt to deal with the interpersonal or intrapsychic problems of the patient, except as they relate to mood," the results have been very good. There are few hospitalizations from the clinic, 73% of the patients are treated without psychiatric contact (except for the initial assessment and medication) and, generally speaking, a cheap, effective, and relatively painless system seems to justify Fieve's subtitle: *A New Model for the Delivery of Psychiatric Services*. We should remember, of course, that drug treatment of affective illness is more specific and more effective than available treatments of schizophrenia.

It is a pleasure to acknowledge the excellent work being done in these and other clinics where mental illness is treated according to sound medical and human principles. Indeed, without their example and the hope that they represent the wave of the future we would not have had the courage to attempt this exposé of practices that we hope will disappear into the same historical dustbin containing the leeches, amulets, and poultices that were the mainstays of the medical armamentarium of yesteryear.

8

The Identity Crisis in Psychiatry

"Anyone can play."
from *Choosing a Psychotherapist,*
—J. Am. Med. Assn.

In this decade many psychiatrists have felt a compelling need to urge their colleagues to *remedicalize* their specialty. Dr. Valerie Cowie, psychiatrist at Queen Mary's Hospital for Children in Surrey, England, believes that the remedicalization is imperative. "We've ignored physiology, ignored organic reasons, due to our blind following of the psychological reasons." She gave the example of autism, now seen clearly to be an organic defect rather than the result of "maternal deprivation."[1]

Dr. David R. Hawkins, summarizing his *Impressions of Psychiatric Education in Western European Specialty Education*[2] stated:

> Although psychiatric education in the United States seems to be more thoughtfully structured and organized [than European], it has overextended itself in an attempt to be too many things to too many people. In many ways, American psychiatry seems to be in a somewhat defensive position, drawing back some of its outposts and regrouping.
>
> Throughout the world psychiatry is having a difficult time metabolizing all the diverse knowledge with which it must deal and seeking to establish its proper function and boundaries.

A growing number of eminent professors of psychiatry, backed by the prestigious report of the U.S. National Institute of Mental Health, have stressed in recent years the biochemical basis of depression, manic–depressive illness, and schizophrenia. In his paper[3], *Observations on the Identity Problems of Psychiatrists,* Dr. Solomon Hirsch, professor of psychiatry at Dalhousie University, puts the problem neatly. "Another component of the identity problem is that some, perhaps many, psychiatrists do not think of themselves essentially as physicians, and still believe that psychiatric illness is largely psychogenic in nature." He illustrates this statement with a description of the successful pharmacological management of two cases.

The first case was that of a teacher who had been forced to give up her work because of agitation and an inability to concentrate. After giving a classical history of endogenous depression, she was subjected to intensive psychotherapy for a year and a half. Her problem was deemed to be penis envy. Her dreams were studied and she suffered guilt in addition to depression when her efforts to understand her "penis envy" were not successful. Later treatment with antidepressant medication brought about a complete remission of her illness. If the majority of the medical profession had allowed themselves similar flights of fancy in attributing leukemia and diabetes to penis envy, insulin would no doubt never have been discovered, and leeching would probably still be in use as a cure-all.

The second case was that of a male physician who had been in intensive analytically-oriented psychotherapy, group therapy, psychoanalysis, and family therapy for about eight years. When he felt that he could no longer go on and became suicidal he went into hospital. "... he quickly responded to antidepressant drugs and was astonished to discover that not only was he no longer acutely depressed, but that he felt better than he had ever felt in his adult life.... "

Although endogenous depression is a clearly recognizeable entity and responds very well to adequate dosage of antidepressant medication, use of these medications demands some skill. The drugs can be used to effect suicide, and patients must be watched carefully in the early stages of their administration. Some tricyclics may cause a bipolar patient to shift from depression to mania, a step from the frying pan to the fire. If used for schizophrenic or schizoaffective patients without being adequately covered by an antipsychotic, the schizophrenic symptoms may become worse.

When all these strictures are taken into account, however, some 70% of endogenously depressed patients will respond favorably to tricyclic antidepressants.[4] Perhaps the percentage would be increased by the monitoring of blood levels and/or the addition of lithium.

On the contrary, according to R. L. Spitzer,[5] the methodological theorist of the American Psychiatric Association: "...psychotherapy is not an alternative to antidepressant treatment and does not prevent relapse or recurrence of symptoms." The excellent response of endogenous depression to antidepressant drugs reveals a record unparalleled in the treatment of other mental illnesses (except perhaps the treatment of acute mania with lithium.) Attempts to substitute ineffective psychotherapy for such a valuable form of therapy are reminiscent of the practices of "conjurors, purificators, mountebanks, and charlatans..."[6] who were inveighed against by Hippocrates 2500 years ago for treating epilepsy by incantation because it was "safe" for the practitioners.

Some psychiatrists wonder whether the profession of psychiatry should exist at all. *The Death of Psychiatry, Help Stamp out Psychiatrists, The Myth of Mental Illness, Demythologizing the Doctor-God, and Shrink,* are titles of recent iconoclastic books and papers written by psychiatrists. The psychiatrists who write them are by no means totally negative about their specialty; in fact, they plead for a remedicalization and rehumanization of the practice of psychiatry through the remarriage of psychiatry with neurology, the use of medication for profound illness, and the provision of meaningful supportive help for the family. They recognize that the first psychological need of a patient suffering from any chronic illness—be it arthritis or schizophrenia, neither of which medical art today can prevent or cure, but hopes to "manage"—is for compassion, understanding, and support from the physician. Naturally the psychiatrists who see schizophrenia as a biochemical dysfunction will be more supportive to patients and their families than those who are psychodynamically oriented and hold patients and/or their families to be the culprits in their illnesses. The latter psychiatrists grind in the guilt and blame that families and patients experience under their care.

Dr. M. O. Vincent in his essay[7] *Help Stamp Out Psychiatrists,* asks the psychiatrist to "discourage scapegoating and blaming of others, especially one particular family member, at the time of crisis within a family." He urges his colleagues to maintain *hope* in the family, to discourage involvement with former problems. His plea is in direct opposition to the practice of one psychiatrist on the faculty of an important medical school, who causes his patients to "experience the pain" of former events. The patients "must not be allowed to avoid painful parts of past experience." Another psychiatrist in the same community has stated that his major therapeutic technique focused on "pounding and punching." His patients are required to "exaggerate" their tensions. Both psychiatrists have expressed the need for soundproof rooms, and one might legitimately, if ironically, conclude that every abreactive (scream) therapist would appreciate a padded cell as a birthday gift.

Another psychiatrist has solved personal identity problems by withdrawing to a nonmedical institute based on the Esalen model. We shall call it "Burning Hills." This doctor had the honesty to withdraw from payment on medical plans and now receives all income from "Burning Hills" which, in turn, depends on fees from clients. This doctor professes to be under the influence of astrologers and spiritualists, welcomes the experience of occasional "possession," participates in seances, works on myths, and gives courses in encounter and related fields. One consequence is the shedding of all responsibility for individual patients, who now must take on "their own responsibility." Many physicians, from the time of Hippocrates to the present, would challenge the view that any physician has the ethical right to abrogate responsibility for the welfare of a patient.

The wholly imagined parallel case in which a physician tells a suffering arthritic patient to take personal responsibility for this illness lends credence to Dr. Ian Hector's question whether psychiatry with its nonmedical treatments would indeed be able to "continue as a recognized medical specialty." Professor Thomas P. Hackett of the Harvard Department of Psychiatry poetically predicts[8] "... that psychiatrists, should they continue winging their way through the heady atmosphere of nonmedical conceptual and theoretical models, will soon find themselves an endangered species." As for himself, "I have felt compelled to keep as much abreast of general medicine as I can in case the worst happens and psychiatry is reduced to the status of phrenology by third-party payers." Perhaps the courageous stand the Burning Hills psychiatrist has taken in dropping classical medical practice entirely would at least relieve the taxpayers of the financial burden on the community incurred by certain of the psychotherapies, even if they are no more effective in the "Burning Hills" environment than they are in the medical office or hospital.

In this identity crisis for psychiatry, some psychiatrists seem prone to delusions of grandeur. Dr. H. P. Rome, a former president of the American Psychiatric Association, declared[9]

"Actually no less than the entire world is a proper Catchment Area for present day psychiatry." He was referring to the social problems of the world that would one day be solved by psychiatrists.

As it happens, many psychiatrists are already abdicating their role as primary therapists to psychologists, social workers, nurses, and others. One might speculate on the cause of this phenomenon as follows: The psychiatrists are trained in, and believe in, psychogenic theory and psychotherapy as treatment for mental illness (see Dr. Hirsch).[10] They have also begun to see that their treatments are notably ineffective. Ergo, they feel they may not be delivering traditional psychotherapy very well and should perhaps call in other types of professionals who may have a better touch.

If this is their mode of thinking, they commit, at a minimum, two errors. In the first place, if psychotherapy is the proper medical treatment for mental illness, then it behooves the psychiatrist as the senior medical specialist in the field to learn how properly to administer this therapy and to remain active in the legally obligatory role of primary therapist. Any surgeon whose patients routinely died under the knife and who thereafter called in the local barber to perform this surgery would receive short shrift from the medical profession. However, the real flaw in the trend to introduce other professions into the role of primary therapist is that psychotherapy is demonstrably ineffective and even harmful.[11] It has no place in mental hospitals regardless of who may be practicing it.

How can we say that psychotherapy is ineffective when the literature abounds in papers demonstrating that psychotherapy results in improvement in as high as 70% of patients? In the first place, the nature of the patients' illnesses is usually not clearly stated. Second, improvement is judged by the same team providing the psychotherapy. By contrast, the National Cancer Institute will not accept evidence of beneficial effect from a proposed cancer treatment unless both diagnosis and improvement are verified by two physicians who are in no way involved with the team performing the research, and this in a field in which improvement is far more objective that it is in psychiatry. But the main fallacy lies in the lack of controls; that is, no comparison is given with patients who are not subjected to psychotherapy. In mental illness (and especially with neuroses, which are most frequently treated with psychotherapy) as in other illnesses, time itself is healing, and if anything positive can be said of psychotherapy, it is that it consumes time.

One of the few *controlled* experiments to test the efficacy of psychotherapy in the treatment of hospitalized schizophrenics is reported by Dr. Philip May, Professor of Psychiatry at UCLA.[12] Of five matched treatment groups admitted to the Camarillo State Hospital, one received psychotherapy, and a second, milieu therapy—that is, room and board and the opportunity to make use of the hospital facilities. There was little to choose between in the results for the two groups and, in fact, the psychotherapy group remained in hospital an average of three weeks longer than those given no treatment. The ECT group showed a better effect while the best results of all were exhibited by patients placed on phenothiazines. The addition of psychotherapy to the drugs produced no additional improvement.

But psychotherapy cannot be written off as only useless. It can also be dangerous. Dr. F. H. Lowy of the University of Toronto has cautioned that we should not "administer psychotherapy without realizing the possibility of negative results, but in effect, it is not done. After all," he quipped, "who publishes negative results." Perhaps as is suggested in the literature of the seventies, anxiety over malpractice suits has kept psychiatrists from frankness about the possibility of negative outcomes with psychotherapy.

The crisis of identity of the psychiatrist may be observed in his blending into a "team". This has been described by Marcus in an essay entitled[13] *The Psychologist as Primary Therapist.* The skills of psychologists are not medical, for they have not attended medical school, but their aptness in behavior modification and biofeedback is lauded in the article. "We were interested to see whether the psychologists could indeed function effectively as primary therapists and what effects the participation of the psychologists would have on the unit, until then so traditionally medical." The psychologists were to learn to participate in determining the type of medication immediately necessary for the patient. The article goes on to say that "within a short time, the psychologists were each carrying four to five patients, a number equal to that being carried by the residents." What justification the authors could dream up for attempting to involve nonmedical personnel in decisions about medication defies the imagination.

Perhaps at this point we might mention the thoughts on "Teams" that research psychiatrists fear will expose patients to inadequate care and create a serious risk of malpractice liability.

Dr. Alan Stone has stated[14]: "The attempts of psychologists to seek parity with psychiatrists in hospitals is simply one more example of their self-determination to pursue economic self-interest in every possible direction. Psychologists obviously lack the medical training necessary to take primary responsibility for the diagnosis, admission, and treatment of patients in hospital. Hospitals will be exposing patients to inadequate care and creating a serious risk of malpractice liability. The American Psychiatric Association should take a stand against this and any other attempt by nonmedically trained persons to assume medical responsibilities to the detriment of the patient."

Dr. Terry Burrows, a Toronto family physician agrees.[15] The Psychologists' Act (which demands a legal status that would enable psychologists to treat patients without a referral) "is a grandiose and paranoid fantasy... a knee-jerk grab for repression and control." But what both Drs. Stone and Burrows have overlooked is that attempts to install psychologists as primary therapists is not entirely a one-sided effort of the psychologists to take over territory previously reserved for medical practitioners. As we have seen in *The Psychologist as Primary Therapist,* some psychiatrists are aiding and abetting this role-blurring process in what we conceive to be a state of confusion about the true role of the psychiatrist.

The comment of the authors of *The Psychologist as Primary Therapist* is: "Perhaps to Dr. Stone's chagrin, they (the nonmedical primary therapists) indeed have responsibility for diagnosis, admission, and treatment." Dr. Stone would undoubtedly be chagrined to hear this rather amazing statement, not because it refutes his worries, but because they would undoubtedly be intensified by the knowledge.

Dr. Melvin Sabshin did not mince words. He concurred with Dr. Seymour Kety of Harvard: "Teams are finished." Dr. Sabshin argues with passion for the remedicalization of psychiatry, the addition of more and better *medical* training within psychiatric residencies, the retention of the role of the psychiatrist as primary therapist, and the abandonment of the anti-intellectual, antiscientific devotion to words rather than facts that characterized psychiatry at least until 1972. He calls for widespread peer review, closer interaction of psychiatry with neurology (not psychology), and a change in the nature of the relationship with consumer groups.

Here is an illustration of the "Team" approach in operation. On another ward of the same hospital from which originated the article, *The Psychologist as Primary Therapist,* a young man admitted himself as a patient, fearing that he would commit suicide. He appeared to become more cheerful during the first four or five days, but later deteriorated badly, becoming disoriented, confused, and manic (he had shown none of these symptoms on admission.) It appeared that, without consulting the patient's family or family physician, the hospital "team" took him off two of his medications (including lithium) and drastically reduced a third. When the family asked who had given the order to discontinue the medication, the nurse replied, "No one person has the responsibility; it was a team decision." A visiting ward psychiatrist later denied this statement and assumed the responsibility. Was this simply an assumption of *legal* responsibility or was he truly *medically* responsible for this fiasco? The incident illustrates the near impossibility of managing serious illness by a team, particularly if the team lacks a clearly designated leader with the ultimate medical responsibility in each case.

As an additional example of role reversal among psychiatric workers, we shall see in Chapter 14, that in a pitifully short stay of six days in hospital before her suicide, Sara Bowdoin, aged fourteen, had as her primary therapist a nurse whose nonmedical treatment was family therapy (stigmatized by Dr. S. Hirsch[16] as a "fad" that psychiatry is "plagued by.") Sara attended group therapy sessions where she was confronted about her thoughts of sex and suicide, plus demands that she fantasize what death would be like. All of this in less than a week. When the nurse spoke of her own qualifications as a primary therapist, she listed her study of suicide. One wonders if she had missed Dr. Alan A. Stone's paper,[17] in which he states "I have presented case material which I think demonstrates that psychotherapy can precipitate suicide or serious suicide attempts." It has also been suggested by Dr. Dorothy Tennov that interpretation of suicidal elements in a patient's dreams, associations, or fantasies cause a risk of actually suggesting the idea to the patient. For this reason, and others, Dr. Tennov feels that the "calculated risk" involved in psychodynamic therapy should be explained to the patient, thus returning us to the ethical concept of "informed consent."

Ms. Bowdoin asks, in Chapter 14, "Did the constant questioning of Sara on suicide contribute to her death?"

A discussion of the identity problems in psychiatry itself would be incomplete without an examination of those roles that members of the psychiatric community feel they should be assuming. We have already mentioned the psychiatrist who took up "possession" and seances as his mode of therapy, and we have seen physicians abdicating their primary role to psychologists, nurses, and social workers. What do all these "people helpers" feel they should be doing for the benefit of the patients?

Some answers to this question may be guessed at by noting the type of continuing education indulged in by this group. Very recently I attended a three day workshop on *Provocative Therapy: Experiential Workshop,* given by Frank Farrelly, A.C.S.W. Attending were two psychiatrists, a general practitioner, four registered nurses including a faculty member in nursing, a psychiatric nurse, and others. The gist of the workshop was that *cures* could be obtained, not only of maladaptive behavior, but also of serious mental illness, including schizophrenia, by honesty that may be brutal in its challenge, insult and even mortification of the patients. A large measure of agreement was obtained from the audience, most of whom were involved in patient care. "I tell my second year nursing students, if we call the patients 'ass-holes' and talk about them behind their backs, and since they come across as 'ass-holes,' they should be told it to their face." Martin Gross, in his book *The Psychological Society*[18] satirically gibes that to cope with such therapists and practices "The truly good patient must also have the ability to talk dirty or the willingness to learn how to." We might add that such a patient would have no difficulty in learning so fine an art from the participants in Farrelly's workshop.

A second participant stated that when she comes to work, she has to be herself. "If I feel angry, I act that way." She does her thing, and devil take the hindmost. Gone are the days when the staff was there for the benefit of the patient! Now all the psychotherapeutic personnel are equal, and moreover, all have the same, or greater, right to express any type of feeling as do the patients. Recently a male psychiatric nurse was encouraged to sue for assault a psychotic patient who had come to hospital via commital. The patient had been driven beyond her slim endurance by the nurse's continually following her around and attacking her self-esteem. When he murmured to her "It must seem terrible that no one likes you," she belted him on the ear. The psychiatrist-in-charge encouraged the suit on the grounds that it would teach the patient responsibility. No admonition was delivered to the nurse for his constant battering of her feeble ego.

To return to our account of the workshop, the lecturer, Frank Farrelly was actively referring the participants to his book,[19] *Provocative Therapy,* in which people are cured of their ills by Farrelly's honesty, which includes calling them wops, Jew bitches, ass-holes, and worse. The attending university faculty members are dutifully buying copies to recommend to their students. A participant vies with the leader to establish who can call the patients worse names. One unfortunate male nurse sadly complains that he cannot do confrontation. This unexpected shred of humanity is attacked by the suggestion that he was probably ineffective in his life as well as his work.

When Farrelly described a cure of schizophrenia by calling the patient a "Yid-kid" who missed his mama, one of the psychiatrists present asked, "You mean their behavior is voluntary?" "They turn it on and off to suit their purposes," answered Farrelly. There was no dissent from the assembled audience.

So let us look at the roles. The nonmedically-trained social worker is here lecturing to the collected nurses, psychiatrists, psychiatric nurse, etc. Is he speaking about the traditional role of the social worker in looking after the needs of patients, in supplying them with housing, good food, companionship, and medical care when they need it. Regrettably not, rather he is discoursing on a personal brand of psychotherapy that includes verbal and scatological assault. The psychiatrists, humbly seeking knowledge, are asking him for an explanation of the nature of schizophrenia. The nurses, far from helping cultivate the nurturing role that their professional title implies, are explaining how they use the hospital to do their thing, and how they call a spade something worse. The one nurse who is apparently guilty of treating his patients the way we believe, and hope, that patients should be treated apologizes for his spinelessness.

Bad dream? Bad joke? Alice in Wonderland?

None of the above. We have just participated in a living tableau on the identity crisis in psychiatry.

9

Psychotherapy is Forever

Patricia and Martin Norman are English. They were married as soon as Martin graduated in engineering. He joined a large engineering firm and was soon known as one of the up-and-coming young men in the field. He and Pat had two children, and the whole family became very much involved in church and community activities. Fifteen years later Martin was offered an excellent position with the Canadian branch of his firm, and he accepted readily. His parents had recently emigrated to Canada, and he looked forward to joining them. The change also gave him a chance for a fresh start since, in the last few years, he had been subject to bouts of depression and self-doubt and had been criticized for the quality of his work. Once settled in Canada the Norman family became involved once more in church and community, but Martin's problems did not disappear magically.

When Patricia was first interviewed she explained how her husband's problems gradually took over the family's lives.

> *Question:* I'd like you to tell me how long Martin has been seeing Dr. Ellis and a few details about his visits.
> *Pat:* Martin has been seeing Dr. Ellis for six years and Dr. Ellis has witnessed what I feel to be a complete breakdown of Martin's personality. He consistently refused to deal with Martin on a medical basis, but instead attempted psychological and family treatment. When I expressed real concern that Martin needed something else to get him through his deeply depressed

moods, his answer was, "I don't believe in medication." He then turned to Martin and asked, "Do you want something?" and Martin, of course, picking up his cue from the doctor said, "No, I don't want any medication."

Question: What was Dr. Ellis's diagnosis of your husband's illness?

Pat: He never gave us a diagnosis. And not only that, everytime I asked for one he chuckled and said, "Would you feel better if there were a name to this?" and I said, "Yes, definitely I would feel better," because I thought there would be some parameters, you know, for me to function inside of.

Question: Were your children called in by Dr. Ellis?

Pat: He wanted both the children there at the therapy sessions, but I didn't allow it, because I realized that although Martin came away all buoyed up, whenever I was at the therapy sessions it was a very distressing situation for me for days afterwards. So I refused to allow the children to come because I felt it would be very disruptive within the family rather than curative. Dr. Ellis was very angry with me for this.

Question: How were you involved in Martin's treatment?

Pat: Oh, in so many ways. They laid out very detailed plans for Martin's therapy in which I played a strongly functional part, but always in a supportive role—I should say a super-supportive role. In fact, I was told point blank at one time that I would have to function for a period as father and mother while he functioned as one of the children of the family! And I was not to feel that this was an insupportable role for me if I really cared about him!

Question: Do you feel you can talk about the relationship with your husband?

Pat: I think so—but where do you start when you're talking about a lifetime with someone? You know, we have a very sensitive relationship and it was just taken apart right from the bedroom down to the shopping center, and somehow it always came out that whatever role I was playing at a specific time was undermining Martin, and that it was up to me to be adaptable, to

> reverse this role structure, to be more supportive to Martin, while Martin should dump his role and take on mine.
>
> *Question:* When you said your relationship was exposed right down to the bedroom, did you mean that you were asked to discuss your sex life with the therapist?
>
> *Pat:* Oh yes. Quite intimately, and not only our sex life—how I functioned in the community, how I functioned as a mother, all those things that I felt I, well—how do you express it? I had felt that I was giving a great deal to the community—and to my family through the community—but all these roles were being questioned as being not supportive of Martin, but directly the opposite. They twisted my life so that anything that built up my own self-esteem—or my reputation if you like—was directly challenging Martin's maleness—his—his potency.

Pat is here voicing a complaint about psychotherapists that has been made by numerous critics. Dr. Sue Stephenson of the Department of Psychiatry of the University of British Columbia has stated, "Psychiatrists are being trained in theories which are hopelessly out of date. It's still being taught, for instance, that a woman's true nature is that of a happy servant and that any form of aggressive behavior in a woman is 'sick.'" Freud attributed all woman's strivings, goals, emotions, and attitudes to penis envy and his disciple, Alfred Adler[1] stated "the feminine sex is inferior and by its reaction serves as the measure of masculine strength." The essence of the scorn that Freud showed for women's achievements is well shown in his *New Introductory Lectures on Psychoanalysis.*[2]

> People say that women contributed but little to the discoveries and inventions of civilization, but perhaps after all they did discover one technical process, that of plaiting and weaving. If this is so one is tempted to guess at the unconscious motive at the back of this achievement. Nature herself might be regarded as having provided a model for imitation, by causing pubic hair to grow at the

> period of sexual maturity so as to veil the genitals. The step that remained to be taken was to attach the hairs permanently together, whereas in the body they are fixed to the skin and only tangled with one another.

Even admirers of Freud would have to admit that the description in these terms of a monumental achievement such as the invention of weaving could best be described as bizarre.

Freud's dismissal of women as developing individuals is expressed in his comparison of the sexes:[3]

> I cannot refrain from mentioning an impression which one receives over and over again in analytic work. A man of about thirty seems a youthful, and, in a sense, an incompletely developed individual, of whom we expect that he will be able to make good use of the possibilities of development, which analysis lays open to him. But a woman of about the same age frequently staggers us by her psychological rigidity and unchangeability. Her libido has taken up its final positions, and seems powerless to leave them for others. There are no paths open to her for further development...

Freud died in 1939, so we cannot excuse him on the grounds of living before the struggle for the rights of women. He had translated works of John Stuart Mill, a champion of the equality of women, but, alas, he somehow ignored Mill's Essay on Women.

Phyllis Chesler has edited a large volume entitled *Women and Madness*[4] to demonstrate that, as Dr. Stephenson states, psychiatrists' view of women is not much advanced from the days of Adler and Freud, or, for that matter, of Aristotle. Pat, had she been familiar with the literature on treatment of women by psychiatrists, would not have been so surprised and shocked.

> *Question:* How did your husband's illness influence your children's lives?

Pat: I'll have to think about that for a minute—there are so many places I could start. Possibly the most destructive aspect of the whole psychotherapeutic process was that by following the psychiatrist's professional advice I was constantly shoring up his theory—and in effect what Martin came to believe too—that most of the trouble arose in our home. The doctor believed that it was a marital and family problem, and when Martin wasn't blaming me, he was blaming his father and mother for the sequence of events in his life—he blamed anyone—his business associates—*anyone* but himself. Even the children began to see that when Martin ceased functioning in the community and on the job, and then lost contact with his parents, the only person he had left to blame was me. And the children saw this consistent blaming—Martin would point it out all the time, you see. He might say: "The psychiatrist said this or Dr. Ellis intimated that if you did this, that would happen, and see! It's happening!" Martin knew that Dr. Ellis considered the family to be responsible for his condition, and he went along with it, just as most patients do—and as most families do—we are *all* so suggestible!

Dr. Ellis did two very damaging things—one to my self-esteem and the other to the self-esteem of Martin's parents. He was very interested in Martin's relationship with his mother and father—you see, there'd been a "role-reversal" in the family, and Martin's father had done a great many things that his mother would have done in a traditional family, and vice versa. Dr. Ellis made Martin feel that this was wrong. And in my own case he made all the work that I was doing in the community, work that I thought was so natural to take up, and a necessity too because it had to be done, seem wrong. He made me feel as though that work was in some way directly threatening to Martin, and I'm sure he made Martin feel this, too. And somewhere or other the very things that Martin had gone to consult him about were lost sight of. Martin's own problems dimmed to obscurity as he dealt with his parents' problems and with my problems.

That's one horrifying effect of those years that I'm unhappy about. But what I'd especially like recorded is my complete disagreement with the approach to psychiatric care adopted at City Hospital, and most particularly by Dr. Ellis's whole department. You see, I hadn't really wanted to take part in those therapy sessions, but they had been set up for us through our minister, who had decided that this was a marital problem. So when we went in to see Dr. Ellis it was already established that this was a marital problem and not simply a problem of Martin's alone—not a problem of mental depression that he'd been struggling with for years, and not a problem of continuing failure at work. Everything had been arranged before I came to the first session, nor was I aware for the first few sessions that Dr. Ellis's office contained a one-way mirror. No one had told me, no one ever said to me that behind that one-way mirror were several—one occasion as many as six—young psychiatric interns from the school of medicine at the university. No one told me that all those minute details of our lives were going to be bandied about by medical students.

Question: If you had been consulted, would you have given permission?

Pat: Absolutely not. I would never have made free with that kind of information in those circumstances.

Question: When did you find out this was being done?

Pat: I discovered it by accident because the room on the other side of the mirror was lit up once. At that point I was alone with Dr. Ellis because he wanted to hear my opinion of the events that Martin had been discussing with him. Martin would have two sessions alone with him, and then we'd have one-half hour session together, and one-half hour where the doctor would speak with me alone. And it was during one of these latter half-hour sessions that I found out that I was being observed. So I asked him "What is that?" and he told me. And I said: "Do you mean that you have been allowing people to view and listen in on these sessions and record *my* feelings when I am not

> even a patient?" I had come there of my own accord to discuss my husband's problems and there they were, without my permission, recording my responses even more carefully than Martin's!

When Patricia complained to the civil liberties organization about the one-way mirror used during interviews with Dr. Ellis, they requested an explanation from the doctor. He replied in part:

> In this teaching setting young clinicians... gain experience, under supervision, in interviewing and caring for patients. At times a videotape is made so that the tape record may be replayed and the various points in the interaction reviewed and discussed. When this teaching procedure is followed the sequence of events is explained and a consent form is signed. On the other hand, when it is deemed appropriate to have students take part in the interview process without being in the room, the one-way screen is used. At this time, the procedure is thoroughly explained to the patient and with verbal consent the interview is carried out. The students then have an opportunity of discussing significant aspects of the interview with the clinician involved. Here there is no record and no signed consent is requested.

Both Patricia and Martin deny vigorously that consent was sought or given.

> *Question:* What was happening to your homelife during these years of therapy?
> *Pat:* Well, on the surface things appeared calm. I mean, no one outside the family knew what was happening. And we did things much as we always had—went for holidays—went to church—the children went to school....
> *Question:* When was the next real disruption in your lives?
> *Pat:* There had been earlier ones before we emigrated to Canada, but the first bad one there occurred one fall.

Martin's father had decided to sell the shop and retire, and we held a party for him at his shop and invited all his customers to come, you know. I was really busy with mum making everything nice and preparing food—and it was pretty late into the evening when I realized that Martin hadn't come. When we closed the shop, his mum and dad came and sat up with me, but I sent them home around midnight. That was Friday. Martin didn't come home on Saturday, or on Sunday, and finally I just couldn't sit waiting any longer. I phoned Dr. Ellis and I told him my fear that Martin might complete a suicide attempt. He had already attempted suicide about twelve years ago and at that time the psychiatrists had said: "Martin, there's nothing wrong with you except that you're lazy! Just get off your ass and get to work!" I was afraid that Dr. Ellis would say the same kind of thing but this time the answer I got was: "There's no need to really worry about Martin. He'll be all right! Just be concerned about yourself and the children." When I pursued the problem further, because I wanted to know where could I possibly get help to find out where he was and what he was doing, he asked: "Do you want to pursue this relationship?" I stood there hanging onto the phone in stunned silence, and I can vividly recall thinking: I'm concerned about a human being's *life*, not a relationship at this point—a very unsatisfactory conversation—

It was several weeks before I heard from Martin. He wrote a long letter to Dr. Ellis and sent me a copy, and I could tell he was screaming for help—I phoned Dr. Ellis and said, "What do you think of this letter?" and he said, "I think Martin is very dramatic! He pictures himself as a nineteenth century romantic hero. He's inclined to be very self-indulgent and very impulsive. So he indulges in impulsive behavior and when he's caught out and has to account for it he runs away." And *that* was all the advice I got from him. I was just supposed to forget about Martin, go on with my own life, and forget about him. But I knew Martin would continue in this impulsive behavior, and I would still be expected to pick up the pieces afterwards.

> What I feel most strongly about after thirteen years of watching Martin go through psychotherapy, and being intimately involved with it, is the terrible waste of human energy, energy poured into a process that has had no proper conclusion. All along I knew that the treatment was unsuited to helping with Martin's problems. It wasn't treatment of any sort—it never got *near* to being treatment. In fact the reverse was true. The effect on myself and on the children was devastating. We lost the creative energies of our normal productive lives, and I consider that we were and are normal productive people. Our problems always had to be centered on Martin's psychotherapy and Martin's changes of mood.
>
> If only he had been given some kind of medication—I fought to have medication, and was told it was old-fashioned, that people didn't believe in it anymore, that it was chemically destructive. And Dr. Ellis would turn to Martin and ask him if he wanted medication, and of course Martin would say no because he knew that's what Dr. Ellis wanted him to say. When I look back on it, I think that it's barbaric that our family has suffered in this way in the twentieth century from lack of medical treatment. Of course, blame is such a terribly useless thing. In all of human behavior there's probably been nothing more damaging than the word "blame" or the action of blame and guilt. That's what happened in our family, and it left the children and me with the terrible feeling that nothing we did to support Martin could ameliorate all the blame and the guilt that we've been made to feel—for some reason that's never been adequately explained to me—

Recently, Martin was at long last introduced to antidepressants and showed a startling improvement, but by that time he had been programmed into believing that his problems were psychological instead of biochemical. Unable to accept such a simple answer to his problems, he refused to stay on medication and as a result he continues to fall into destructive depressions. Only the threat of permanent separation from his wife forces him to return to medication from time to time.

Diabetics go into coma from metabolic imbalance when they drift off their medications, and high blood pressure patients have strokes when they don't take theirs. Similarly, not every case of mental illness that *can* be managed on medication has a happy ending. Martin's case does not end happily because he is what is called noncompliant with the medical regimen. Seven years of mistreatment programmed him to refuse to accept proper treatment when it was offered to him.

The question of "overservicing" or what one might call "soliciting" is raised in the treatment of Martin Norman. He suffered six wholly unproductive years of psychotherapy under Dr. Ellis, a process that also involved his wife and might have involved their children if Patricia had allowed it. She submitted to the sessions on the understanding that her presence was necessary if Martin was to become well again. Dr. Ellis was displeased that the children were not involved since his preferred theories demanded that the entire family attend the therapy sessions.

Many psychiatrists must view anyone who enters the office as a patient, which was certainly Dr. Ellis's approach to Patricia. She was asked the most intimate questions about her emotional and sex life in a psychotherapeutic atmosphere that demanded frankness. Since her personality is a reserved one, she suffered considerably from this invasion of her privacy. One of her objectives in the present interview was to alert other women not to permit themselves to undergo this kind of demeaning experience. Although Patricia has great inner strength, she feels the therapy damaged her self-esteem. Dr. Ellis made her feel guilty about her involvement in community affairs. She was made to feel she had neglected Martin whenever she attended conventions, and when she received public recognition for her work it was deemed to be castrating to Martin. Dr. Ellis would only give approval for a supportive role to her husband.

Dr. Ellis' position on the family is not the most extreme that has been taken by psychiatrists. A school exists that believes there is no such thing as an individual patient.[5] What there is is an "index patient" who has been "selected by his family to act out the family pathology.... the patient is thereby only externalizing through his symptoms an illness which is inherent in the family itself; he is a symptomatic organ of a diseased organism."

A psychiatrist at a Sick Childrens' Hospital insists that the entire family enroll at his clinic as a patient before he will treat a child. The family is required to sign a contract that they will remain in treatment. (The contract, verbal or written, represents a frequent invasion of the marketplace into psychiatric practice. For example, a young woman left in her suicide note the statement that she was sorry she had broken her contract with Dr. Wyle. Apparently, Dr. Wyle had felt that the contract was sufficiently strong medicine for suicide prevention that no antidepressant medication was required.)

Patricia's belief that the demeaning family "therapy" to which she was exposed was unproved is substantiated by recent reviews. A recent NIMH publication[6] reports that "a lack of appropriate methodologies have led to major difficulties in efforts to substantiate the concepts [of family therapy]." An article in Journal of Family Counseling[7] presents a critique of the field of marriage and family counseling, especially the paucity of empirical research related to therapeutic outcomes.

Dr. Ellis refused to consider diagnosing Martin and in fact chuckled when requested to. This attitude is widespread among many echelons of psychotherapists and is, of course, in keeping with their thesis that the patient is not suffering from a real illness, but from some sort of aberration or perversity.

In truth, diagnosis is one of the cornerstones of medical progress. Diagnosis serves at least four major useful functions. First, it provides a shorthand description of the disease so that, within broad limits, one can understand what the patient's symptoms and signs are likely to be. For example, the statement that a person is a juvenile-onset diabetic tells us that he or she has likely lost weight, drinks a large volume of fluids, passes a great deal of urine, and may have come to hospital comatose or semicomatose with certain fairly specific signs. Second, the diagnosis suggests the treatment; acute appendicitis suggests surgery. In such a case, incorrect diagnosis may mean the death of the patient. Third, the diagnosis suggests the prognosis or outcome of the disease. Patients with infectious hepatitis ordinarily recover completely, but a small percentage develop chronic hepatitis or cirrhosis of the liver. In the fourth place, clinical research and statistics are impossible without accurate diagnosis, since it becomes impossible to determine what is the natural history of the disease or the effectiveness of treatment if it is not certain what disease is being treated.

Much of psychiatric literature is bedeviled by inaccurate diagnosis. For example, the American penchant for overdiagnosing schizophrenia[8] initially made it very difficult to determine which segment of the population of mental patients would benefit most from lithium since too many people with affective disease were so diagnosed. This caused a great deal of overlap in the results of therapy on what were supposed to be two distinct groups of patients, but actually represented two mixtures. The problem is partly one of greater difficulty of diagnosis in psychiatry than in other branches of medicine. Such a difficulty, however, should be a challenge to improve diagnostic accuracy and not to chuckle at the foolish patient who would like to have a diagnosis.

Elsewhere we have discussed the advances that are being

made in using reaction to drugs and family history as aids to diagnosis. But much improvement is possible within the traditional framework, and DSM-III[9] will apparently sharpen the diagnosis of the major mental disorders by laying down a number of necessary and sufficient conditions for the diagnosis of each disease. For example, the existence of hallucinations will no longer score a point in favor of schizophrenia *if* the patient is at the same time strongly manic or depressed. This restriction is a recognition that anyone with an active mental illness, and not schizophrenics only, can hallucinate and that only prolonged hallucinations without major affective disturbance suggest schizophrenia. In any event, a physician who refuses to struggle with the problem of diagnosis cannot be considered to be a physician.

To return to Martin and Patricia. We really cannot say whether or not Martin was a treatment failure for medication since he has not taken his medication consistently enough to enable a decision to be made. Let us say he was a treatment failure.

The negative effects of drug treatment failure do not begin to compare with the disastrous disruption wreaked by the unquestionable treatment failure of seven or more years of psychotherapy. Not only was Martin taught to shift blame for his problems to anyone in the vicinity, but his relationship with his father and mother was permanently severed. That his wife, who was subjected to years of humiliation and worse at the hands of Dr. Ellis did not also desert him owes to her faithfulness and love, and is only little short of miraculous. The children were partially protected from the same destructive process by the courage and good sense of Patricia.

Perhaps nothing worse can be said of psychotherapy as it is usually practiced is that drug therapy, with all its inadequacies and side effects, is generally less painful, less harmful, even when it fails.

It may be objected that none of the excesses of psychotherapy are as dangerous as the worst side effect of phenothiazines—tardive dyskinesia. This possibly is true. However, even those over-fifty patients who are at risk for tardive dyskinesia do not develop the disease until the drug has been used for many years. A drug that fails to produce benefits is discontinued after perhaps three months—12 months at the longest, thereby eliminating any possibility of TD.

Psychotherapy is forever.

10

Treatment by Incarceration

Dorothy Smith was the elder of two children. Both her parents worked. She began experiencing severe depression shortly after she had graduated from secondary school, although she had had some trouble earlier.

Her mother was interviewed.

Question: What was your first experience with a psychiatrist for Dorothy?
Ms. Smith: When she had just graduated from high school. She refused to go to junior college, or to university, or to any vocational school, or even to go out and get a job. She just wanted to sit at home. She didn't want to see people either. I felt she was showing signs of what looked to me like depression and I felt she needed help. So I took her to a person who was recommended to me as "the very best".
Question: Who was that?
Ms. Smith: That was Dr. Locke. He had seen Dorothy some years before when she had been having difficulty attending school, but at the time she had not wished to continue with him. After she left him she grew better, and so things went along reasonably well until after she graduated from high school. But when she seemed depressed again and unable to function, I took her back to him.
Question: Did he put her on medication?
Ms. Smith: No. And he told me that I must not allow her to manipulate me, that there was nothing the matter with

her, and that what I should do was insist that she leave the house. He said that this would force her to do something. We were very reluctant because she didn't want to go, and she begged to be allowed to stay home. I couldn't just put her out into the street, so I made arrangements for her to move into the YW; then on the day that she was to move I came home from work to find that she had taken an overdose of some pills and though she was not in a coma, she was very drowsy. I tried to reach Dr. Locke and was told that he was in conference, and that it was simply impossible for him to speak to me even though I had made it clear that it was a real emergency. When I sent through a second message, I was relayed a message that I was to take her to the Emergency Room at the hospital, which I did. I waited there for over an hour for him to come. In the meantime they had pumped Dorothy's stomach and she was all right again. When he finally came, he told my husband and me, "This is further manipulation. You do not allow her to come home. You lock the door and you insist that she carry through with the original plan."

Dorothy went back to the YW, but in a few days phoned her mother to say that she had decided to kill herself. Her mother brought her home again. Ms. Smith knew there was no point in returning to Dr. Locke for help, and therefore attained a referral to Dr. Metz. He had a reputation for using a common sense approach to young people's problems. After interviewing Dorothy, he prescribed heavy medication. Dorothy, however, firmly believed that her problems could be solved at home. So she refused to take the medication he had prescribed and she refused to attend interviews with him. Finally, Dr. Metz told Ms. Smith that Dorothy must be hospitalized.

Question: Why did he want Dorothy to enter hospital?
Ms. Smith: Because she had refused to take the large doses of medication he had prescribed for her, and she wouldn't go to see him. When I questioned forcing her, he said that I was denying her the chance to develop her own

strength. He said that she was in the condition she was in because I had always overprotected her, and that the only way she would recover would be if we forced her into hospital and she *had* to learn to use her own strength. At his suggestion, we did not discuss hospitalization with her. She was simply tranquilized heavily and taken to the regional mental hospital in an ambulance. When we went to see her there, she pleaded with us to take her home, and she continued to plead for all the months she remained there. But the doctors always insisted that she had to stay there if she was ever going to get better.

Of course, as soon as Dorothy entered hospital, Dr. Metz no longer treated her. As a rule, psychiatrists don't continue with their patients once they're in a mental hospital. They are assigned to a staff doctor instead. And I have come to think that anyone who is very ill suffers a traumatic experience with any change in doctor. Furthermore, at that hospital the doctors are exceedingly busy. I've forgotten what the last figures were, but certainly they spend fewer than fifteen minutes a week with each patient.

Mind you, I really liked Dr. Gartner whom Dorothy was assigned to. I felt he was a caring person, that he genuinely wanted to help her, and that he did his best. But I think he was entirely ignorant of the conditions that existed on the ward.

Question: What were those conditions?

Ms. Smith: The patients were usually left alone on the ward while the staff stayed in the nursing station. Physical conditions were dreadful; the beds couldn't have been more than two feet apart. If patients didn't want to get up in the morning, they were forced to. I was told that Dorothy was manhandled. The patients were herded to a huge dining hall where the staff stood and watched them eat. No effort was made to create a caring or pleasant atmosphere. You could pick up the feeling of hopelessness as you entered. Patients paced up and down, some shouted and ranted.

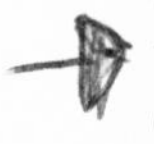

The hospital in which Dorothy was incarcerated (the word seems just) is one where the nurses had the power to put patients in solitary for punishment without doctors orders. On one occasion, a young man was shipped down to the hospital from upstate in a very agitated condition. He was immediately placed in solitary, where he hammered on the door to be released. Six hours later he was found dead of a lung hemorrhage consistent with viral pneumonia. Another patient had his nose fractured by a male nurse because he would not sweep the floor. Other patients who witnessed the attack were not permitted to testify because "it would not be in their best interest." (Cf. the suit brought against the patient in City Hospital because she boxed the ear of a male nurse who followed her around telling her how unloved she was. On this occasion, the suit was brought "in the interest of the patient" in order to teach her responsibility.) Another patient was scalded to death in a tub. Still another, in an excited phase, was resisting an order and being taunted by a male nurse—he was held down by four male attendants and smashed in the mouth with the loss of two teeth. No appointment was made with the hospital dentist and the incident was not even included in the discharge summary! The widespread allegation of mistreatment of patients in California Mental Hospitals culminating in numerous deaths at the hands of staff is now history.[1]

Question: Do you mean Dr. Gartner wanted her to stay in hospital longer?
Ms. Smith: Yes, for her to stay there, although she was very unhappy and begging us to take her out. And he refused to see her, to recognize her feelings, and to recognize the fact that she was not getting better. She was, in fact, getting worse. I was able to talk to him once a week, but that was only because I had figured out the workings of the hospital and I was able to—well, I simply phoned very early every Friday morning to talk to him. Other parents and families never see the doctor at all. But

while Dorothy was in that place no one ever listened to her—including me—and I felt guilty about that for a long time...

Question: Did she get the medication Dr. Metz wanted her to have?

Ms. Smith: I have no way of knowing. Many of the doctors in mental hospitals or wards consider that the patients' families do not have the right to know what treatment their children or relatives are getting. We asked what Dorothy was getting, but were told that we would have to leave that to the doctors. A friend of mine—a radiologist whose daughter was in the same hospital—had to leave the city for a few weeks. A colleague of his called the hospital to ask how the daughter was doing and made the mistake of asking what medication was being used. The surly response from the psychiatrist was "If you think you can do better than I can, take her out."

Question: Then you didn't have family conferences with this doctor about Dorothy's illness?

Ms. Smith: No. I often begged him to see all of us together to explain the treatment, why he insisted on her staying in hospital against her will, because I felt that the rift between us was widening. We had been led to feel that she was deliberately being difficult and I'm sure she had been made to feel that we didn't care about her. As I look back I realize that if I had only had the strength, I would have said, "No, this is my child. She needs time and she'll be all right. And I will try to understand her the way she is and accept her the way she is." But I listened to these "experts"—you see, when I originally trained as a nurse, psychoanalysis was in the ascendancy. All the brightest young doctors were either going to be psychoanalysts, or thought that psychoanalysts had the answer to all the world's problems or were undergoing four to seven years of analysis themselves. We all seem to be learning the hard way that it just isn't true...

At last, Dorothy's family realized that her health was deteriorating, and arranged for her release. She returned home in time for Christmas. Two months later, she took her own life. She was nineteen years old.

> *Ms. Smith:* I feel very definitely that my daughter's death was caused by her imprisonment in that place. That sounds like a melodramatic statement, but there is no doubt at all that her experiences there made her feel that she was a very sick person who would never be well again, and never function happily. She told us this in her farewell note to us, and I know that she felt she could never hold her head up again because she'd been in there. The whole milieu, instead of helping people to get better, only makes them feel worthless, crazy, useless, and hopeless.

After Dorothy's death, all members of the family suffered great distress. Ms. Smith was haunted by the thoughts of what she should have done or said to help her daughter. She visited Dr. Metz to discuss this and the doctor promply told her that it was obvious that she needed hospitalization and major tranquilizers. Ms. Smith comments on this below:

> *Ms. Smith:* I think a good deal of harm is done to people who go to psychiatrists, because psychiatrists see all the people who come to them as "sick people." But frequently they're just troubled people, people who have experienced unusual stress of one kind or another. What they need is support, and they need encouragement to use the strengths they have—the strengths that they've been using for years. Temporarily these strengths have been undermined because of a stress situation. This was the case with me.
>
> I believe that what I was expressing was normal grief over Dorothy's death. I think that you always have a choice with people who are grieving—whether you let them find the strengths that have enabled them to function before, or whether you immediately move in and manipulate the situation.
>
> *Question:* Did the psychiatrist give you a choice?
>
> *Ms. Smith:* No. But I realized I had a choice. It was a

choice of accepting the label of sickness that he wanted to place on me, or saying to myself: "Look, this has happened to you and you have to deal with it the best way you can. Going into hospital isn't going to help you now. As a matter of fact, it will be very damaging for the people who need you." I think everybody has this choice. I know there are times when the stress is so severe that a person might need help for a while, but for that help one need only see a general practitioner, or a priest, or a friend. It's terribly important that psychiatrists understand that they must give only as much support as is needed for grieving people to keep functioning and that they encourage the "well part" of you that's always there, temporarily overwhelmed perhaps, but always there and always able to be brought to the surface again with the proper kind of support.

Question: Would you recommend the services of a psychiatrist to other people?

Ms. Smith: No. I would never go back to a psychiatrist myself. And I wouldn't recommend that anyone else go, except someone who is temporarily or chronically suffering from a chemical imbalance—and then I would be very careful who I went to because I don't believe that *all* psychiatrists understand the use of medication in treatment. Perhaps a good internist or GP would be better.

Not all women in Ms. Smith's predicament have been able to see that they had a choice. Ms. Palmer's son was sixteen when he began experimenting with drugs. Within a year, he had a "bad trip" and wound up in the emergency ward of the general hospital. When his immediate medical needs had been dealt with, he was referred to a psychiatrist. Dr. Marks promply diagnosed the boy schizophrenic.

To Ms. Palmer this term was as good as pronouncing a death sentence on her son, and she became very disturbed. Dr. Marks referred *her* to another psychiatrist, who arranged for her immediate hospitalization. There she was given electric shock treatments. Ms. Palmer went in and out of hospital for the next five years, and was constantly and expensively involved in psychotherapy. At last, the psychiatrist decided that she could function independently and she was discharged as "cured." A few months later she took her own life.

What happened to her son? He is now an insurance salesman and functions with no medication whatsoever. There is considerable doubt whether the psychiatrist's diagnosis of his condition had any validity at all.[2] Several papers have shown that schizophrenia is diagnosed many times more often in North America than in Europe and England. Perhaps the stricter diagnostic criteria set out in DSM-III, if adopted, will reduce this discrepancy.

It is very tempting for some individuals to respond to psychiatric soliciting as Ms. Palmer did. Ivan Illich[3] warned of the tendency "to make people abdicate their healthy ability to deal with suffering." It not only proliferates the number of patients unnecessarily treated to their probable detriment, but it is also costly, whether paid for by a medical plan or by the patient.

Dorothy's mother was convinced that her imprisonment in the provincial mental hospital had caused her death. Other parents also tell of the dehumanizing environment in large government institutions: On three consecutive Sundays, Mr. and Ms. Evans went to visit their son who was a patient in one. The first week they were told that he was "out on the grounds"; they searched the grounds for him, but were forced to go home without seeing him. The next Sunday they were told the same thing; they searched and again left without completing their visit. On the third Sunday when they were told he was "out on the grounds," they looked in the ward instead. They found him in his bed, lonely, and disconsolate just as he had been on the two previous Sundays. Mr. and Ms. Evans wanted to tell the administration what they thought of this willful cruelty, but they feared their complaints would make their son's treatment worse. He had previously told them that the staff cursed at him and humiliated him for being fat. The parents felt helpless.

One parent, however, risked all to improve the conditions of her daughter's hospitalization. She wrote a letter to the director of the hospital and sent copies to her family doctor and to the Ministry of Health. Among her "requests" was this one: "that you will please ask the nurses (especially the one named Lorna) to stop telling my daughter that she is a parasite and likes being sick. She is very ill and depressed, and it may not be possible to abort her next suicide attempt as was done last Wednesday!"

It is very strange that in all other specialities when the patient is hospitalized the doctor intensifies his care and concern, but that psychiatric patients are abandoned by their doctors when they enter a mental hospital. In *Psychiatry at the Crossroads,* a report prepared by a task force from the psychiatric section of the British Columbia Medical Association, it was recommended that "each patient should retain his own individual physician through all phases of his illness." Apparently, the profession does sporadically realize the inadequacy of the situation, but to the present date no steps beyond this recommendation have been taken to rectify it.

When Dorothy Smith was in hospital Ms. Smith asked her daughter's psychiatrist to meet with the family. Ms. Smith thought that if they could meet, the hospital psychiatrist might then explain his treatment plan so that the whole family could understand and accept it. Supportive and compassionate help from a physician is necessary for any family to confront and attempt to understand an illness serious enough to require hospitalization. Dorothy's family was never granted the single session asked for, though we are all too well aware that other psychiatrists are happy to intimidate whole families into attending therapy, or weakened spirits such as the unfortunate Ms. Palmer, into entering hospital.

Dr. Ian Hector, when chairman of the Board of Examiners in Psychiatry for the Royal Physicians and Surgeons of Canada, has remarked on the psychiatric residents' lack of ability to develop a safe, sound informed plan for treatment. They could give no plan for the management of suicide except hospitalization, and were really unable to discuss planning and implementation of a plan for treatment... "We cure rarely, we should comfort always." Comfort, in the case histories in this book, has been rare.

Dr. Hector stated that psychiatrists may find themselves trapped in a dogmatism "divorced from the clinical reality of the sick or distressed person." This dogmatism was seen in Dr. Locke's treatment of Dorothy as a "manipulative" person who should be locked out of her home. Such patent cruelty originates in psychoanalysis itself and is a theme stressed by Dr. Kurt Adler, the son of the famous Freudian. He speaks of the "privileged position" of the depressed person who feels "superior" and "forces" people around him into his service. Perhaps Dr. Adler sees few hospitalized patients, and has no empathy with their agony. Far from "forcing people around him into his service," depressed patients receive shock treatment against their will and are denied visitors they long to see.

The book and film *One Flew Over the Cuckoo's Nest* gives the literary lie to this hypothetical imagery of the mental patient "manipulating." The patient in this epic was constantly harassed by the staff, given shock treatment that was not indicated, and finally had a lobotomy performed simply because he was independent and would not go along with the system.

"I had 128 ECT. There was no way for me to get out of it. They took my clothes away, rolled them up in a bundle and tied them up. I didn't sleep all night, and then waited in a day room until I was put in a little cell with a bed at 8 AM with one sheet over my shivering body. I heard other patients choking and gasping for breath. The nurses are used to fear. They watched me shake. One man hid in the bathroom, but they found him and dragged him to the ECT room." This from Marlene, an ex-mental patient and journalist who never recovered from the psychic trauma—the forcible exercise of an excessive amount of ECT against her wish. Who is manipulating whom?

Many lessons could be drawn from these cases.

First, the isolation from community, relatives, and friends that typically occurs when a patient is admitted to a Mental Hospital must be abolished.[4] "The individual exists in his most naked, lonely, anxious, defenseless state when he is ill and hospitalized . . . he is . . . increasingly surrounded by a faceless technology that separates him from the outside. Hope often seems remote, while at the same time previous abstract considerations of life, death, and dying become concrete." To mitigate this disastrous break with the continuity of the patient's life, it should be legislated that such patients cannot be denied visitors of their choice. Families and friends, far from being barred from councils discussing the patients' welfare, should be enlisted as the most valuable allies, as is routinely done at the Clark Institute of Psychiatry's Schizophrenia Clinic.

The referring physician should make a practice of visiting the patient regularly. Physicians and staff who hold the philosophy that the patient is "manipulating" them or otherwise voluntarily misbehaving should be re-educated in modern medicine, and if the education process fails, they should be removed relentlessly from the system and replaced by humane, scientific, and empathetic staff who will try to help the patients over this most severe emergency of their lives, rather than making it more difficult for them.

Patients must have the right to know what their treatment is and will be and, under all feasible circumstances they, or responsible relatives should have to give informed consent, especially to such hazardous and potentially dangerous treatments as ECT, provocative psychotherapy, primal scream, and so on.

Perhaps when these, and other recommendations in a similar spirit, are introduced, we will see a happy synthesis of modern medical practice with the beneficial "moral treatment" of mental patients that was so effective and humane in the 19th century instead of the combination of the 18th century punitive methods with 20th century psychiatric fads that is only too often practiced today.

11

The Family is the Patient

> The parent who gives the
> child love and concern can
> still have a mentally ill child.
> That is the tragedy of being a parent.
> —Dr. Louise B. Ames

Marilyn Hendricks has three younger siblings. Her father is a fireman; her mother a clerk in a department store. As with most families in the suburb where they live, a good part of their income goes to making monthly payments on their house mortgage and on their car. Most of the financial worries and the problems of raising their children seemed behind them, when Marilyn, at the age of fifteen, became ill.

Marilyn, an unexceptional high school girl, began to lose interest in food and gradually spoke less to her friends and family. She finally refused to attend school. After she had lost thirty pounds from malnutrition and dehydration, and became totally uncommunicative, her parents were finally frightened into taking action by the following incident, described to us by Ms. Hendricks shortly after it occurred:

> I was about to leave for work one morning when I went into the bathroom looking for some Kleenex. I found Marilyn standing there, unclothed, unspeaking, and apparently unseeing. I tried to get her back to bed, but she

> just remained there, unyielding and immovable. Since I had to get to work, and I assumed she would become cold and return to bed, I left. Jim had already taken the children to school and left for work.
>
> When Jim returned from work seven hours later, Marilyn was still standing there! Although up till this we had been trying to think that she was just passing through a phase, we now realized she was seriously ill and sought medical help in a hurry.

Marilyn's presentation was unusual, and resembles what was called in Kraepelin's[1] classical description of the four predominant types of schizophrenia "catatonic stupor." Although catatonic patients were rather rare—representing perhaps 2% of the total schizophrenic population—they had been extensively studied because of their inherent interest, and because they presented certain distinctive biochemical abnormalities that were recognized as long ago as 1938.[2] The catatonic was often biphasic, like the manic-depressive. In the phase of catatonic excitement, they might be mistaken for a manic patient, except that they were even more excited, if possible, and more bizarre. The catatonic stupor was unlike anything seen in depression. The patient might sit for hours or days in a stereotyped posture—head thrown back or eyes cast down, one arm perhaps elevated. A peculiar wax-like immobility is described, in which a hand could be lifted by an observer and would remain in the new position for hours or even days. No response could be obtained, by word or gesture, to any communication. The patients often died within weeks, but if they survived an excited or a stuporous state, they might have periods of complete or partial remission, only to relapse again. Gjessing found that the biochemical abnormalities in the blood and urine of these patients were the same in the excited or stuporous state, which is the reason for the term catatonia being applied to both, even in patients who only show one manifestation.

As is true of other of the more flagrant forms of psychosis, catatonia may be becoming even rarer than it was. It is also being found (a finding that is also not confined to catatonia) that a patient may present as a catatonic, or with catatonic features and, after one or two attacks, settle down to a more garden variety of schizophrenia, or, indeed, undergo remission.

Marilyn does not answer to the complete classical description of a catatonic. Her presentation was close enough, however, that it would seem reasonable for a psychiatrist who was acquainted with the history of the voluminous research on the disease to attempt to make the simple biochemical measurements that would establish her similarity to or difference from Gjessing's classical cases. We shall see that a different path was taken.

Marilyn was quickly referred to the psychiatric ward of City Hospital, where she was given six ECT and afterwards placed on a short course of medication. Neither the referring doctor nor the Hendricks were ever able to find out what medication had been administered although they tried persistently. Marilyn told her parents she had received blue pills (Stelazine, an antipsychotic, comes in blue tablets), that they made her feel better, and that she wanted to take them.

The psychiatrist in charge of Marilyn, Dr. Farris, decided after ten days that Marilyn's illness had been caused by parental discord and abruptly discontinued the medication. In accordance with a widespread practice among psychiatrists, he decided that "family therapy" was the correct treatment, even for a condition whose biochemical basis is becoming ever clearer. The entire family—Jim and Mary, Marilyn and the three younger children, aged eleven, thirteen, and fourteen—were required to participate.

First, the three younger children were interviewed by a twosome—one male and one female psychiatric nurse. Do your parents fight with one another? How does Marilyn get along with them? Do you and your sister discuss your parents? How do you feel about your father? How do you feel about your mother?

Next, the parents were barraged with questions about their life, including intimate details of their sex life. Marilyn was questioned again and again on her relations with her family. She was asked with which parent she would choose to live should they separate. Marilyn remained mute.

After she had been in City Hospital two months, the Hendricks underwent the psychological trauma of signing Marilyn out. She was receiving no medication and had shown negligible improvement. They feared that Dr. Farris would order the reinstitution of shock treatments, and Mr. Hendricks was worried about the effects of so much psychological probing on the stability of the family. "We have the other three children to keep together, and we don't need the added suffering and suspicion that the family sessions generate."

Dr. Farris warned that Marilyn could never return to City Hospital for help if her parents removed her without his blessing. Similar threats were made to Frank's parents (see Chapter 1) when he was signed out of another hospital in despair at the mistreatment he was receiving. In fact, the threat is a common, although unenforceable, form of coercion used by psychiatrists to circumvent the legal requirement that patients (or their agents) must give consent (informed or otherwise) to treatments. For this reason among others, we feel that the difference between treatment received under voluntary admission of a mental patient and under committal is not as distinctly different as is sometimes thought. A recent White Paper reviewing the British Mental Health Act[3] seems to agree that, although the involuntary committal process in Britain has virtually disappeared, it apparently in some instances has been substituted by a putatively "voluntary" admission, and proposals are made to provide extra protection for such voluntary mental patients, for example, by obligating the hospital to make them aware of their legal rights as they enter.

Now, having removed their daughter from an environment that they felt was doing her no good, and moreover a situation that was injuring the family's coherence, the Hendricks embarked on a quest that is only too common: the search for a compassionate and competent physician who would provide effective help for their disabled daughter and who also would not add to the already heavy burdens imposed on the family by the child's serious and incomprehensible illness. The route taken by the Hendricks was to approach a general practitioner, who then referred Marilyn to a community care team. The team psychiatrist arranged for her admission to the pediatric ward of a district general hospital for a few weeks evaluation. Here, the story of City Hospital was repeated with a few variations. Marilyn was again put on medication—this time, the use of phenothiazines was not kept secret—and began to improve. However, she suffered some bouts of postural hypotension from the drugs, becoming dizzy from low blood pressure when she stood up, and the medication was therefore decreased to a token amount. Marilyn continued to be uncommunicative, apathetic, and extremely slow in her movements, but her nutrition improved.

After two weeks, she was sent down for a few hours a day to the psychiatric Day Care Center attached to the hospital, a facility whose only two activities were group therapy and attendance at the local bowling alley.

Dr. Roberts, the psychiatrist in charge of the Day Care Center, was apparently angered by Marilyn's silence, which he seemed to interpret as a form of misbehavior rather than as a symptom of her schizophrenia. He demanded that she speak, and when she was still silent, he threatened her: "I'm going to send you to Idylwilde [the Regional Mental Hospital]!" Marilyn was sufficiently in touch with reality to be terrified by this threat, and her parents found her quivering when next they visited her. Although they could see history repeating itself, they had really exhausted their options and had to stay with the situation in the hope that it would improve.

The following Monday was Marilyn's birthday, a day for which permission had been granted for her to start a weekend pass at home. When the Hendricks called for her on Friday, she was distraught; Dr. Roberts had revoked the permission. He now thought going home was not a good idea, and he had so convinced the referring physician. According to Dr. Roberts it was not safe to expose Marilyn to so many family problems. At the same time (just as had occurred before the suicide of Sara Bowdoin in Chapter 14), Dr. Roberts was promoting the idea of early discharge of Marilyn so that she could live at home, from which she would then attend the Day Care Center. The inconsistency of his position makes the denial of the long-awaited weekend pass appear more of a punitive than a therapeutic measure. Of course, Dr. Roberts may have felt that he was putting pressure on Marilyn to improve her behavior, or that he was practicing behavior modification; more likely, he was simply oscillating between a number of theories, as the psychotherapeutically inclined often do.

Mr. Hendricks spent the afternoon talking with his daughter, trying to soften the blow and calm her fears. She was very anxious, feeling that she had not been allowed to go home because she was about to be sent to Idylwilde, where she knew she would be on a large ward with many more seriously disturbed people, where visits from her parents could be severely curtailed, where she could be put in solitary confinement at the whim of a nurse. Although Mr. Hendricks endeavored to reassure his daughter, his reassurance was not very credible, because he, himself, was not certain whether Dr. Roberts had the power to execute his threat. He also asked Marilyn whether she agreed with Dr. Roberts that they were a bad family and did that add to her worries? In her turn, she reassured her father and added, "Other kids think I've got a pretty good family."

The following day, the parents were called to a conference attended by Dr. Roberts, Dr. Yerkes, a psychiatric resident, a worker from the Day Care Center, Marilyn, and the referring physician.

Mr. Hendricks said later, "My wife and I felt we were on trial whenever we met Dr. Roberts. Marilyn did too, and always felt unusually agitated when she knew she would see the psychiatrist. Dr. Roberts asked every sort of question about our lives before we were married—*personal* things—right in front of Marilyn. But I finally drew the line. I told him we had been all through that at City Hospital, that Marilyn left there in as bad condition as she had entered, and that our family life had nothing to do with her illness. My wife and I had a good relationship and we were not going to be crucified again."

The Hendricks were not, as were some of our unfortunate interviewees or their families, the type who went to the library and read everything that had been written on the subject of the illness that had struck a loved member of the family. They were, therefore, unaware that they were fighting, and partially winning, a war that had been going on for at least thirty years between the adherents to various schools of "family therapy" and the parents and relatives of mentally ill children. Does this sound rather a far-fetched exaggeration? Let the "family therapists" speak for themselves.

In the beginning, there was Frieda Fromm-Reichmann to whom is attributed the concept of the "schizophrenogenic" mother: "dominant, rigidly perfectionist, lacking in confidence, distrusting, cold, masochistic, low in self-esteem, inconsistent, rejecting and dependent."[4] Having filled thousands of psychiatric journal pages on this concept, the theorists of the "family therapy" movement moved on to define the "schizophrenogenic father," and finally even the "schizophrenogenic family," which is

> "characterized by an excessively punitive and hostile father child relation, parental maladjustments with significant disharmony, greater maternal dependence, and greater capacity in the parents to distort reality to suit personal needs. Schizophrenogenic parents, like neurotic parents, have a need to infantilize the child and perceive him as incompetent..." "The fundamental insight of family therapy and the basic premise of family theory is that the family is the basic unit of conceptualization. The patient is thereby only externalizing through his symptoms an illness which is inherent in the family itself. He is a symptomatic organ of a diseased organism."[5]

Some of the descriptive epithets applied in the literature to the unfortunate father of a schizophrenic child (implying, also, a causal relationship) are

> "relatively uninvolved in the family life except to punish or give financial support, weak, immature, passive, totally inadequate in fulfilling his family role, cruel, sadistic, domineering, hostilely dependent on his wife, distant... and brutal."

Although the quotations date from 1964, they are given in extenso because they appear in a massive review article with 130 references, all playing variations on the same theme: namely, that the schizophrenic is no different from any other member of the family. The pathology belongs to the family and the schizophrenic is merely indicating it. In fact, he or she has been chosen for this role, he or she the "index" patient, the "identified" patient.

Lest it be thought that we are flogging a dead horse, we find little change in more recent references. A book published in 1976, called *Family Therapy: Theory and Practice,*[6] brings us up to date. "A number of fascinating publications, mostly recent, and mostly American, have tried to show that families cause, or help to cause one of their members to be schizophrenic, and some of these claim to show mechanisms by which this terrible subjugation takes place." The conclusion to this discussion, expressed somewhat wistfully, is "An etiology so elegantly worked out should eventually lead to a basis for treatment, but as Henry Massey and I showed in an earlier paper the family theory of schizophrenia has neither been well developed in practice nor had much demonstrable success." As our own case histories have shown, this lack of demonstrable success has not discouraged "health care team" members from inflicting the "elegance" of their concepts of the "domineering, brutal, passive, sadistic, masochistic, schizophrenogenic" parents (and siblings too) on those unfortunates who have turned to them in their despair. The psychiatric resident who first treated Frank (see Chapter 1) expressed a wish to bring the whole family into hospital, while the chief of the service informed the family that Frank would never get well while he lived in the same city with his family. James Framo, professor of psychology at Temple University, the triumphant victor in a three year struggle to set up a Family Unit within a community mental health center writes in 1976[7] that symptoms are faked, selected, shared, carried vicariously for someone else. The family "designates" the patient, often assisted by well-meaning, but naive health care professionals. Professor Framo feels that one of the major roles of his unit is to find out if, indeed, there is a patient as such (other than the family).

In 1964, Meissner said, "We must not forget the other members of the family, the so-called 'well siblings.'" With startling originality, we find Framo enumerating in 1976 the advantages of evaluating the "so-called 'well' sibling." Note the shift in quotation marks.

Bruno Bettelheim makes physical use of the family theory in his "therapy" of children who are too young to understand its verbal expression. Outside his Sonia Shankman Orthogenic School for Psychotic Children sprawls a twice life-size concrete statue of a nude "supermother," which the patients are encouraged to attack, kick, stomp on, paint, and scrub.[8]

The attack on parents as the cause of mental disease in the children has not been confined to the parents of schizophrenic children. For many decades, the standard theory of childhood autism postulated that it was caused by a particular type of parent. As long ago as 1943, Professor L. Kanner described[9] a stereotype of the parents of autistic children in similar terms to those of Meissner and Framo. His description was expanded upon and converted by later writers into the cause of the illness with devastating effects on parents already reeling under the burden of adjusting to and caring for a child suffering from what is probably one of the most distressing diseases known. In 1969, Kanner publicly denied ever having claimed that the parents *cause* the disease, which he described as "innate."[10] "I hereby acquit you parents." Very kind of professor Kanner. When one recalls that one of us became interested in this problem as a result of the suicide of the mother of an autistic child, Professor Kanner's acquittal seems very similar to the "rehabilitation" of executed political prisoners in a totalitarian state after a shift in the ideological breeze.

Professor Bettelheim has not rehabilitated the mothers. His fantasy about the autistic children "glued to hate" because they were "thwarted or ignored" in early childhood of the love they craved lays a mantle of heroically tragic proportions on the shoulders of small, brain-damaged children, and an infinitely heavy burden on their parents. Dr. Bettelheim finds, we know not by what means, "hatred, extreme and explosive, and behind that hatred was always the longing, eternally thwarted, but nevertheless never given up; a longing now deeply encapsulated in repression so as to keep it from coming to awareness in unbearable pain."[11]

Bettleheim is sure that the mother's personality characteristics caused the disease. Kanner now denies this, but believes that he gave an empirical description of that personality. That the whole issue is again one of reading preconceived notions into the situation is suggested by recent research carried out with more attention to reasonable scientific norms, which shows that there is no truth to the Kanner-Bettelheim stereotype. The parents of autistic children turn out to have the same spectrum of personalities as the parents of normal children.[12] If there is a small excess of emotional disturbance (not proved), it can easily be attributed to the strain of living with an autistic child. Thus decades of self-recrimination, guilt, and anguish suffered by the parents of these damaged children were based on the "elegant" exposition of a piece of bad research. Jim Hendricks wrought better than he knew when he counted himself out of the proffered "family therapy."

Having persuaded Dr. Roberts that his family demanded a different type of solution, Jim asked for a conference on future treatment for Marilyn. In the course of the discussion, Dr. Yerkes, the resident, remarked on the cramped quarters of the Day Care Center and proposed that Marilyn be transferred to the University Teaching Hospital, which had ample facilities for the physical activity that she had been lacking for so long. Dr. Roberts disagreed; if the Hendricks did not care for Idylwilde, the Day Care Center would do just fine.

Marilyn was then discharged home with appointments to return to the Day Care Center. Not surprisingly, she refused to attend, and the burden of her management again fell on this working couple. A beneficial legacy of her recent stay in hospital, however, was the provision of an interested social worker who realized that Marilyn was not involved in a therapeutic situation. In an honest attempt to take a forward step, but held still partially in thrall by the family theory, she suggested a "parentectomy." Marilyn should be moved to a boarding home, away from the influence of the "noxious family." So Marilyn was moved from her comfortable home with its surrounding familiar faces to a strange environment, where the meals were not of the best, where the overworked staff had little time for her, and where she again lapsed into silence and partial immobility. But she was not as immobile as she had been, for one rainy midnight she tiptoed out of her shared bedroom and started to walk the ten miles back to her home. As Christian Beels, speaking of similar coerced separations, put it, "They seem to have a way of getting back together again."[13]

All too often these charades recur until the parents, broken by a tragedy that they seem unable to mitigate, half convinced by the "therapists" that the child's illness is indeed their fault, finally allow their children to be sent to the Idylwildes and Glenhavens, where they may or may not receive reasonable treatment, and where they may still spend long portions of their lives. We met a well-to-do couple at a resort who had committed their son to the State Mental Hospital and had been convinced that it was in everyone's best interest that they not see him. Their grief and guilt resulted in the husband's early retirement so that the two of them could travel together, obliterate their pain in alcohol and, like the Ancient Mariner, seek a sympathetic ear into which to pour their story.

With the Hendricks, it was different. Stubborn Jim would leave no possibility unexamined. He discussed the problem with his dentist who had had a schizophrenic patient. The patient came from a small town fifty miles away and the only psychiatrist there seemed to be quite different from those described by Mr. Hendricks. He seemed to believe that schizophrenia was caused by a biochemical dysfunction of the brain and that it needed to be treated with drugs. He was no advocate of "magic by mouth," and his first sentence to the parents of his patient was, "This could not have been your fault."

Jim and Marilyn immediately traveled to visit him; fifty miles was nothing after the struggle they had waged. Dr. Harman admitted Marilyn to the medical ward of the small hospital where he practiced, and settled down to the consistent application of modern psychopharmacology. In ten days

Marilyn was well enough to go home with Dr. Harman's prescription. No fear that she would not follow it. "Daddy, he gave me the blue pills that made me feel better at City Hospital."

A year later, Marilyn, still on an adequate dose of phenothiazine, is again becoming a functioning member of the family. She does her share of the housework, is in good physical health, and works part time. We ran into her quite coincidentally in the emergency department of a local hospital where she had taken her younger brother to have his leg stitched up. We could hardly believe that this tall, smiling, friendly young woman was the same mute, impassive person we had seen a year earlier.

Marilyn has not yet returned to school, but hopes to soon. She has not recovered completely, and may never, but she is rehabilitated to the point where she and her family can live with her disease. Best of all, Dr. Harman's simple and inexpensive treatment has proved to the satisfaction of the Hendricks that she is suffering from a physical illness, and that it was not their warped personalitites that had caused "this terrible subjugation."

With so gratifying an outcome, it becomes easier for us freshly to contemplate some of the sadistic terminology used by certain theorists of "family therapy." Burton L. White, director of a gigantic research project at Harvard on the development of the personalities of pre-school children, is quoted in Life Magazine,[14] "The mother is right on the hook, just where Freud put her." Since Freud himself never used such inelegant language, one wonders what simile Professor White is thinking of. To us, the picture is of the worker in a blood-stained apron hanging a carcass on the hook of a slaughterhouse assembly chain.

Thomas Szasz, a psychiatrist who is noted for his irreverent attitude toward most of the sacred cows of psychiatry, seems to agree: "Family therapy—I call it family butchery."

12

The "Identified" Patient

Alix Williams is the third child in a family of four. One older sister had died at the age of five, long before Alix was born. Her father is a building inspector; he is a sensitive man who has good rapport with young people and has worked for many years with his church's youth group. Alix's mother, Sonia, does volunteer work among senior citizens and at the local art gallery.

Alix was fourteen when illness struck. "She was well on a Wednesday, in increasing confusion on Thursday and Friday, worse on Saturday, and on Sunday she would have crossed the freeway and not even known the cars were there." She confused what was real with what she imagined; her thoughts had become disordered. She was terrified by experiences that existed only in her mind. Whenever she was rational she agonized about slipping back into unreality. "I'm going crazy, mom!" she would say.

Sonia Williams related the following:

> *Sonia:* I phoned our general practitioner, who sent us to a psychiatrist. It was the beginning of a strange new life for our family. Our privacy was totally invaded, but we were quite willing to go along if it would help Alix.
> *Question:* Who was the first psychiatrist that you saw?
> *Sonia:* That was Dr. Mason.
> *Question:* What was Dr. Mason's diagnosis of Alix's illness?

Sonia: He didn't give us a diagnosis. But he did things and said things that in retrospect I found shocking and outrageous. At the time I felt that since he was the specialist, he knew what he was doing. He was totally into the sex bit—one of the things that he did that I now find repulsive was to show her a variety—many, many, pictures—of animals in various stages of copulation! Now for Alix this wouldn't be too shocking because in our house we've read everything, we go to shows together and discuss anything and everything, but for some children who are not exposed or who have been sheltered, this would have just been terribly surprising and shocking to them.

Question: What was Alix's reaction?

Sonia: She just very sanely explained it to me—I was not present at that session—she explained what he had done. She thought the whole thing was quite ridiculous, and yet at that time *she* was considered insane!

Dr. Mason wanted to know every detail of *my* sex life, or lack of it, because I was married at nineteen to my love, and I'm still with him and that's it. He couldn't believe it, you know, that seemed abnormal to him. Alix said, "Mother, do you think he wants to have an affair with you? He keeps asking me if it's true that you've never had an affair with anybody."

Question: What was Dr. Mason searching for?

Sonia: I haven't the faintest idea. Maybe Alix was right. But my husband and I decided that this was all so far out that we didn't take her back again. It was nearly the end of June then anyway, and we went on a family holiday. We really believed it would help Alix, but it wasn't more than a week after we arrived at the resort that she had to be hospitalized. Dr. Bentley was the psychiatrist.

That was her first experience in hospital. My husband and I stayed right there with her for four months and the rest of our children returned to the city. But before they went, we were all brought together in Alix's room and Dr. Bentley was there and Alix leaned toward me—she was very, very ill at the time. Her hair was long and untidy—and it fell across her face several times. I pushed it to one side, stroked it, and I felt that this was the most normal thing in the world to do. But later, when Dr. Bentley talked to us, the hair situation was the thing that he picked up on and he said that this was a most *abnormal* thing to do, that you'd only do it to a small child. I was bewildered by his reaction, but I just could not agree with it.

When we felt that Alix's condition was stable enough, we brought her home again.

Question: How long was it before you needed professional help again?

Sonia: When she was sixteen. This time the psychiatrist was Dr. Renton and he also asked us to come together as a family. We rather liked him. He was mild in appearance and manner, but later I was always astounded to recall how much power this man had over us. He would lean back comfortably in his chair, smoking his pipe while we on the other side of his desk were in so much agony. On our family visit, only our other daughter was missing, because she was out of town. As part of the questioning routine, we were asked to move around the room, just to walk around and then, when he said to stop, to stand with someone. We did this, and the boys stood together, my husband moved beside me or I moved beside him, I'm not sure which, and the doctor immediately said, "There's the answer! Alix has been left out of the family!" For my husband, this was the most terrible thing that happened to us throughout all the psychotherapy that was done. He still thinks about that. He finds it indescribably terrible for the image to remain with Alix that she was an outsider.

Question: What was the reaction of the other children to this?

Sonia: Oh, at the time they were quite willing to do anything they could to help her. But I think that when they look back now, they realize it was nonsense and didn't serve any purpose. But, you know, I think they grew suspicious of everyone's motives, especially in the family—for quite a few years. You see, during the course of all that psychotherapy—I remember using the phrase "the opening of Pandora's Box"—we were always being asked to search for every negative, unhappy, painful incident in our family history having to do with Alix, or between one another in any way, shape, or form. Nobody ever asked what was *good* about our family, what was positive! He never tried to use the numerous family strengths to ease our suffering.

Question: Well, just for a minute let us talk about the family's positive features before we return to the painful happenings in your lives. I believe you had a very happy family.

Sonia: Yes, this is so true, and the saddest thing for me is that we have come close to forgetting all those beautiful years before Alix became ill. In summertime when my husband's work took him out of town, we went along, and the six of us were together all summer long. It was just one long picnic. We saw just about the whole of this region. And at home the children were in clubs—and their father and I were so involved—we really loved each other...

You know, I remember Alix came home one day—she was in outpatient group therapy at the time—she said that today they had all been questioned about their families. Most of them apparently were saying that they just hated their families, and that's what they expected Alix to say. That was the right answer. But Alix said, "No, I don't hate my family. I love my sister and brothers and my Mom and Dad," and the rest of the group told her, "Then you really are crazy!"

Question: Who was the doctor at that time?

Sonia: That was Doctor Davidson. There was another time—I was not there, but this is Alix's story. She'd said it very clearly and she's said it many times, so I believe that it's true. Dr. Davidson said that the best time for her family was when she was most ill because her illness drew us together and therefore made us more of a compact unit with an ill member of the family to work for, but when she was well, then there were problems in our family. And that's an oversimplification—and it's totally wrong!

You know, our eldest died of cancer just before she was five—Wilm's tumor of the left kidney. She lived for five months after her illness was discovered and we nursed her. We had her at home almost the whole five months. But what we remember most about that time is that everyone was so compassionate and kind. Doctors, nurses, relatives, neighbors, friends—there was an outpouring of love and concern that surrounded us and supported us and it was all love, no blame. I remember later reading in the paper about children who had accidentally taken poison or had been in a car accident, or whose father backed a truck over him in the driveway, and I used to think, "Oh, how terrible!" because these parents had to take the blame-and when our daughter died of cancer, I thought there could be nothing in our lives worse than what we had just been through. I should have known better. With mental illness there is a special feeling of having been singled out, not to mention the out-and-out accusation, from doctors and nurses and from the other workers whom you meet. Discord is sown within the family. Your neighbors and your friends have a field day psychoanalyzing you and your whole situation. There must be a reason, they say. I really wonder what goes on in their house! They can't be the loving, happy family we thought they were! All of this gets through to the patient and family. Freud and his followers have programmed the thinking of this world, and this *must* be changed.

Question: What did you mean by out-and-out accusations?

Sonia: Oh, there have been so many. At one time we thought of putting Alix in a group home, and one day when she had an appointment with the doctor, I went over to one of the cottages where she was to live with a group. I went in and explained to the man there who I was and why I was there—that I had wanted to see the physical place and its feel. He made me very welcome, brought me a cup of coffee, and sat me down. Then he went to get his superior, a young man, a social worker, who came up to me and said—I can still hear his rough voice—"Why are you here?" And I told him that the doctor had suggested that Alix should live in one of the cottages and I wanted to see what they were like. And he said, "No wonder your kid's sick with an interfering mother like you!" I've never forgotten that, because if I hadn't taken an interest they could just as easily have said, Humph! Uncaring parents, no wonder she's ill! So it was damned if you did and damned if you didn't—but that's what happens to the parents of children who become mentally ill. I think my intellect takes over somewhere here and I *know* that people like him are wrong. What bothers me is that other parents are going to him and his kind today, and will tomorrow and the next day if something is not done very soon.

Question: Most of your experiences with psychiatry are negative, Ms. Williams.

Sonia: Oh, please don't let me convey the image that I'm hostile and bitter toward all psychiatrists and their support staffs. When Alix went into hospital that first time, the nurses there were beautiful to her, and one in particular I remember because she gave me something that was really valuable and I still keep it with me. I'd been saying to her, you know, this is going to happen and that is going to happen, because I was already programmed to think the worst, and she said, "How can you possibly know?" And I said, "Well, we've been through this at home several times already." And she said, "You couldn't possibly manage this at home; it's a twenty-four hour a day job. We go away from this after eight hours totally drained, totally exhausted!" And we got talking and then she said to me, "Now don't quote me on this, or I'll lose my job, Ms. Williams, but people like you put doctors on a pedestal and don't question what they do, and you don't trust your own common sense. And that's wrong. Doctors do make mistakes." I really have to thank that girl for that, because sometimes, when the weight of my daughter's illness and the way it was being treated have almost broken me, I regain the perspective she projected for me and with it the strength to go on a little while longer.

Question: Alix has been in hospital a number of times since then, hasn't she?

Sonia: Oh yes, four times in five years. Four months that first time, three months in the general hospital, one month in our district hospital, and almost six months in the regional mental hospital.

Question: What was the nursing like?

Sonia: In the mental hospital, some of the nurses are very cool, and they don't get involved. But there are a few that I'd really like to thank. They care, you know, and they have just held Alix's hand and put an arm around her shoulders, and they've done more than they had to do. The young nurses who come in, the nurses in training—Alix really relates to them—they make her happy. There are volunteers, and they certainly did work hard and they were very good. But I only saw them at Christmas time.

Question: I believe that at one time you took her to the university teaching hospital for help.

Sonia: Yes. She'd been extremely ill at home. I had been up all night and day with her, and was very tired and asked her father to look after her for a few minutes. It wasn't his fault. She could run like the wind and away she went but I thought I might be able to find her—and I did. Then because I just didn't seem to be getting any help from the doctor we had, I got her into the car—at this point she was high but really clear—and I took her out to the university hospital and I said to the person at the desk, "Somebody just has to help me help my daughter." The charge nurse came over and took us in to see the psychiatrist on duty.

> *Question:* Who was this psychiatrist, do you know?
> *Sonia:* I can't recall her name. Alix was excitable by then. She talked incessantly for about an hour and was questioned. Then the psychiatrist asked the charge nurse to take her away. Alix went into the lounge, sat down, and played the piano so well the doctor simply couldn't believe it was her and she asked, "Is that her?" And I said, "Yes, this happens all the time." And the psychiatrist said, "There is nothing we can do for your daughter here. She is too ill. This is an open ward hospital. She needs a closed ward hospital. Take her home and do your best and the next time she becomes impossible to handle, take her to the emergency ward at the general hospital."
>
> You know, I'm a reasonably strong and capable person, but I can think of many parents—mothers *or* fathers—who would just fall apart at that point and understandably so—because I almost did myself.

Alix is now treated by a psychiatrist who has explained to her family that her illness is a result of her biochemistry periodically going awry. Strangely enough, that diagnosis is precisely the same her family was given the first time she was hospitalized in the resort town they were visiting. The general practitioner who had first examined her said then that this was definitely a psychosis, but that no Freudian theories of interpersonal relationships need be found to explain it. He explained further that it was a biochemical illness that must be controlled by drugs under medical supervision. Regrettably he then referred them to a psychiatrist who was completely committed to psychotherapy and totally rejected medication.

However, Alix is now on combined medication and for periods of time she leads a normal life. She sometimes has a job, enjoys sports, plays the piano, and goes dancing. But the illness breaks through again when, as has sometimes happened, her medication is cut down owing to a communication problem between the psychiatrist and the community team. She then becomes incoherent and disoriented and generally needs to return to hospital.

How have her brothers and sister weathered these years? The youngest boy recently told his mother that Alix's illness hadn't affected his life at all. But then he added that he thought "it had made each one of us keep more to ourselves." The other son has said that "sometimes I wanted to run away as far as I could go," but this is the same young man who has stood with tears rolling down his face when Alix was really ill, and cried out, "Can't they do anything to help her?"

Although she knows that the family did nothing to cause Alix's suffering, her older sister still wonders and feels guilty when she doesn't give Alix enough of her time. She is still haunted by the memory of a visit she made to Alix in the hospital. While there, she had gotten into conversation with several nurses. She asked whether they knew how this had happened to her sister, and they told her, completely convinced of the truth of their pronouncement, that Alix had never been appreciated by her family, that this had caused her illness.

Someone once asked Alix's sister: "When your mom and dad aren't able to look after Alix, will you take over?" She replied, "I don't know. I'm not that big or that heroic."

Alix's father first refused to believe that she could not be perfectly well again. But through horror, then compassion, has finally come a small degree of acceptance of her chronic illness.

And her mother?

> I know it's ridiculous, but I still feel that Alix's illness might not have occurred if I'd treated her differently. I am so programmed to think that. Intellectually I know her biochemistry runs amok, but again and again I fault myself.
>
> It was family therapy that brought out the worst in our family relations. It left scars—particularly with my husband. He is not the same person he was. I feel, and I've

> said it before, that we were left broken and bleeding on the floor and that no help was given to us at all. We had to pick ourselves up and put ourselves back together again—and this is not an easy thing to do...

Sonia's description of the terrible moment when the psychiatrist decided that Alix's illness was the result of having been an isolate is echoed in the stories of other parents.

Gordon's parents had not realized that their son was having difficulties until he came to them for help when he was seventeen. They were a family of very private, restrained, and gentle people who loved one another deeply, took considerable pleasure in each other's company, and had great family loyalty. But they never pried into each other's lives. Since Gordon's personality change had occurred only slowly, the family had taken little notice, feeling that his new reticence resulted from his growing maturity. Now he required psychiatric help, and his parents and siblings found themselves in family therapy, their quiet world battered apart. On one occasion, Gordon's sister was interviewed by the psychiatrist: "Joan" he said, "your brother's problem is your mother. She is over-involved with him. She really hasn't any time or left-over feelings for your father or the rest of you." Joan protested: "But doctor, it's because he's so sick! She'd be just as involved for any of the rest of us if we get sick—and I think she'd have a sleeping bag across the threshold of my father's room if he were in the hospital!" Ironically after a few years had elapsed, Gordon was involved with a new psychiatrist who announced confidently that the root of his problem was his cold, intellectual, detached mother, the same woman who'd been accused of being over-involved.

Sonia Williams' encounter with the social worker who decided in the instant of their first meeting that she was her daughter's problem is repeated in the experience of Ms. Chester, who phoned her district mental health service when she discovered that her middle son was taking drugs and began to fear for his mental health. She explained her problem to Ms. Herrin, the social worker who took the call.

"Who does the boy remind you of?" asked the social worker.

"Well, come to think of it, I guess he reminds me of my brother," said Ms. Chester.

"What do you think of your brother?"

"Well . . . he's a bit of a rotter, I guess. We visit with him in the summertime, though."

"There," said the social worker, "is the answer to your problem. Your son is like your brother and you unconsciously compare them, so that your expectations are that the boy will be a rotter, too!"

Fortunately, the boy outgrew his interest in drugs and is a happy, reasonably well-adjusted member of the family.

Among other burdens the Williams were forced to bear was the concept of the "identified patient." In this model, the patient is "chosen" by the family to act out the family pathology. Dr. Renon illustrated this in the game of musical chairs he played with the family to show that Alix was isolated. It was also his *ad hoc* concept, expressed early in the "treatment," that the family functioned best when Alix had her relapses.

"Did you choose her as a scapegoat?" This is the brutal question left with the fated family. The cruelty of the concept is exceeded only by its futility.

"Family" therapists would have us believe that they have changed their emphasis; that they are now concerned with developing the strengths of the family and in providing support. The Williams case and others in our files suggest that there is a cultural lag between theory and practice.

Because, as far as I can see, the mayhem continues.

13

Anorexia Nervosa

Heather Danes' father is a research scientist. Her mother, who was a graduate of the Sorbonne, was for many years a university lecturer. Her only brother was born three years before her. When Heather was fourteen, her parents were divorced, and although she was of course affected by this always painful event, there was no significant change in her lifestyle. She was an enormously vital girl with an enthusiastic interest in sports, and considerable academic ability. In addition, she was a highly social creature.

Heather began to suffer from anorexia nervosa shortly after puberty. One of the symptoms of her illness was a dysperception of her own self. She saw herself as a fat person and was intent upon starving herself toward what she misperceived as a more suitable image.[1] Heather would eat ravenously—emptying the refrigerator—and then go into the bathroom for self-induced vomiting. She thus gradually began to suffer malnutrition, and wasted physically to the point where she appeared to be little more than a skeleton.

The remainder of her story is taken from an interview with her mother.

Question: At what age did Heather become ill?
Dr. Danes: I should say that her personality really started to change at the age of fifteen when she began to look out of the window in the school room instead of concentrating, and she took to sitting in her bedroom by herself. But she wasn't ill, or at least we didn't recognize

any ominous symptoms at that time. Then when she was almost seventeen, our family doctor referred her to Dr. Peters, a psychiatrist. After a little questioning, he asked her if she'd had sexual relations with a man. She told him she hadn't, so he said that that was her problem and he told her to go out and get some sex! And do you know that such is the power of a doctor's command that she went right out and picked up a young man in a bar! She was brutally seduced, but she stayed in his power for three whole months, trying to effect the doctor's cure.

Not long afterwards, I emigrated hoping for a quieter life. But Heather's school work continued to slip and she became dangerously thin. She wouldn't eat because she was convinced that she was getting fat. Finally when she was just about eighteen, she had to be admitted to the psychiatric ward of the university teaching hospital. She was diagnosed as a classic case of "anorexia nervosa."

Question: Were you involved in her treatment there?

Dr. Danes: Yes. The hospital "team" said that it was exceedingly important for me to go daily. They wanted me to attend interviews with the psychiatrist and Heather, and this I did. I went there thinking I was going to give background information and cooperate with the psychiatrist, Dr. Nelson, but I found that I was being treated rather like a hostile witness! Anything I said was pounced upon and questioned as though it had some hidden meaning, as if it contained some secret that could shed light upon Heather's illness by showing something I had done wrong. I remember on one of these occasions when I had been asked to explain myself, I tried very hard to be specific, choosing my words with great care. When I'd finished, the doctor took his pipe out of his mouth long enough to say, "Words! Words! Words!" After all, how else was I supposed to express myself if I didn't use words? I should have answered, "What did you expect me to do—tap dance?"

The "team" were always asking Heather about her feelings for me—Heather *wanted* me, she *asked* for me. She told them she needed me and that I was the one

person in the world that she could really trust and rely on and that she must have me by her. Over the course of the treatment, they used to encourage the "naughty little girl" side of her to complain about Mommy—petty things, you know, and rather puff them up. After interviews that had taken this turn, she would look at me uneasily, and it was often a good five minutes or so before we reestablished our normal relationship, because they had driven a wedge of suspicion between us. It was really rather ridiculous because what they were doing worked against the patient's declared wish to enjoy the support of her parent. On one occasion Dr. Nelson opened the conversation by asking Heather how she was getting along with me. When she answered, "Very well," Dr. Nelson retorted, "You're very good at hiding things, aren't you?"
Question: How did Heather adapt to the hospital?
Dr. Danes: I don't think she was ever quite sure of her bearings. One of the first things that I remember rather upset her was that the doctor, who had made no mention of this to my face, said to her on several occasions, "Your mother can come to hospital at any time; we have room for her." And Heather, thinking that she was being constructive relayed the message to me and said, "You know, the doctor told me you could come at any time, Mommy, and have a rest!" And I said, "What on earth would I want to do that for? I wouldn't be there for medication. And I couldn't rest in a mental hospital!" She was quite upset because I didn't take up his invitation, because she saw it as a nice rest for me.

Later on, when the "team" talked with us, the female nurse also seemed to be hell-bent on driving a wedge between my daughter and me. Heather and I have a very relaxed and easy relationship, we talk very openly to each other—we don't have secrets from each other and in many ways we're friends as well as mother and daughter. But they encouraged her to complain in a childish way about things that Mommy wouldn't let her do—Mommy didn't like her playing television at three in the morning—and they always saw her side of the question, never mine! They even told Heather—I'd been explaining to her that the amount of food which she ate and then made herself throw up was a strain on my budget—it was a *vast* amount—and I said, "You know, I can't really afford it, and besides it's wasteful." She went and relayed this to the nurse, and the nurse, who has no knowledge of my financial position said, "Oh, but your mother *should* be able to cope!" And Heather came back and told me this as though the judge had passed a ruling. The nurse also said to her, "Your mother should get a job," and this is something the psychiatrist had also said. I didn't consider it any of their business how I organized my private life. I was making tapes for the French Department, doing volunteer work with the senior citizens, visiting my friends, and going for walks to relax when I was worried about Heather, and I felt it was impertinent for them to tell my daughter what her mother should do. Who was the God Almighty ruling that I should do this? A psychiatrist who knew nothing about my life and a psychiatric nurse! I was so annoyed that the next time I was asked to attend the interview between Heather and the psychiatric nurses, I asked this nurse whether she had told Heather I should get a job, and she looked at me in a rather superior way and said, "Yes, I did." And I said, "Well, I think that was impertinent!" She said, "Oh, do you?" And I said, "Yes, and you annoy me, you are so smug!" And she said, "Now what does that word mean to you?" That's really cutting you down to patient-size, isn't it. So I said, "It means exactly what it says in the Oxford Dictionary!"

Somewhat later on in her treatment, we were in a group with Dr. Nelson and the psychiatric worker, Heather and I. Dr. Nelson—he was the head psychiatrist on the ward, by the way—told us to stand up and push at each other's faces. Well, I just couldn't push Heather's face. I simply put my hands on it, and he complained afterwards that I hadn't pushed hard enough.

Question: What do you think he was trying to evoke?

Dr. Danes: I don't know! I thought it was inordinately silly because I guess he was trying to unveil some sort of aggressiveness, and being a rather civilized person I would certainly never have pushed my daughter's face like that even if I'd felt like doing it. In a normal setting I would have no hesitation in showing justifiable anger at Heather if I was provoked. We don't have a repressed sort of relationship at all.
Question: I think most people stop this kind of behavior when they're about five.
Dr. Danes: Possibly you might feel like doing it...
Question: But you usually don't do it.
Dr. Danes: No.
Question: Perhaps you could express how you felt toward the psychiatrist at this time?
Dr. Danes: Yes, I can tell you how I felt. At first I had been very disconcerted by him and then I had become exceedingly resentful of the treatment Heather was receiving since I had tried in every way. I had read about analysis, I had reflected on the history of our family relationships, about things I had done and things I hadn't done to see whether I could find anything there. I came to the conclusion that my family was not essentially different from any other family and that I could not feel any more causal responsibility for my daughter's illness than I would had she developed leukemia or thyroid disease. I think it is cruel, when a family is struck by a devastating illness, and one is doing all in one's power (with no practical professional guidance) to help, to be made to feel that I am killing her.
Question: You wanted to tell me about the care Heather received after her discharge from the hospital?
Dr. Danes: Yes indeed. I was given a glowing picture while she was still in the hospital of the excellently organized aftercare she would get from a community care team. I was reassured over and over because I kept saying I needed assistance with Heather. And they assured me that she would get help. Well, when she came home, it

turned out that the help was not to be daily as we had been told, but just on Monday for an hour, when she would speak to two psychiatric nurses, one male and one female. In addition she had to attend a weekly session which was called, rather gloriously, "group therapy" where a group of outpatients sat around a table waiting for their medication. Some of them spoke incessantly, but others were silent. These were urged to "open up." "You're not being open enough," was the phrase with which they prodded Heather.

Heather went a couple of times and then she managed to dodge this group for three weeks and felt vastly better for it. I forget what pretexts she made, but she arrived, collected her medication, and left. She just dreaded going there, but the doctor insisted she had to go. Sometime later, I talked to him about this after she had told me that she was simply filled with rage whenever she thought about going there. So I *told* him how she felt, and he just said, "Yes, well..." I never got a reaction from him! But on another occasion—she always had a bad evening before having to go to the group—she had to take extra Valium, and on this one occasion she took all of her sleeping pills the night before to avoid going there. She just couldn't face it.

Question: That hospital and its associated community care team promises to help the patient find a place to live and a job after discharge. How did that work out?

Dr. Danes: Once she had come home, she was told by the psychiatric nurse that she shouldn't be living at home, but they didn't do anything about it. She was just left with me.

Question: Didn't they help her to find an apartment?

Dr. Danes: No, not at all. They simply kept telling her she shouldn't be living with her mother. For occupation, which they told me at the hospital was very important—and I agreed—there was a service that provides twenty-five hours a month of work paid at a rate below the minimum wage. I went with Heather to the office where it is organized and the man who interviewed her said, "Oh, I can see you're very artistic. We'll get you a job at the Art Gallery. Yes, I can see by your writing, that you're very artistic!" And we came away very pleased. But it transpired that the job was not a daily occupation of two hours a day, but that it meant nothing for twenty-five days of the month, and then for five days she was expected to go for five hours a day to the Art Gallery, not to do anything artistic, but to stay in a windowless room with large cupboards full of magazines and bundle up these magazines! Well now, she only weighed ninety pounds and she is five feet seven inches tall, and she's very nervous and she found it desperately lonely and exceedingly hard work. By the end of the week she collapsed and had to give it up, having waited all month for it to come about.

Question: Was there a drop-in where she could have coffee or tea and companionship, and perhaps some kind of activity?

Dr. Danes: I believe that at one time they did have some kind of out-patient recreation center at the hospital, but they don't have it any longer. There's only the "group therapy" sessions, which as I told you was a desperately unpleasant experience for her. In desperation, I told the community team that she absolutely needed some sort of day program. I was told that there was one at City Hospital and the nurse from the day team accompanied her there. That turned out to be another great disappointment. The doctor was never there; in fact no one was there the first three times that she tried to join it. In the end I phoned to find out what was happening. I spoke to the worker involved and she said, "Oh, the people don't show up all the time, but when they come we go and play shuffleboard!"

Question: Heather still requires hospitalization from time to time, and no system of management for her illness has been established by the doctors. Are you definitely satisfied in your own mind that family problems were not the cause?

Dr. Danes: Definitely. But then again, although I have consciously rejected this theory that the parents are primarily responsible and having gone back very carefully over our whole life, I feel I've provided an unusually happy home for my children. My son is happily married and successful in his work and family. And yet there's that insidious poisoning which we all undergo that somehow leaves me uneasy—a little, not exactly guilty, but rather responsible. Parents cannot avoid this sort of feeling. The psychiatrist would serve a much more useful role by attempting to allay this unwarranted guilt rather than exacerbating it. I once asked Heather's psychiatrist if he ever said, "This can happen in a happy family." His answer was an unequivocal, "No."

Question: Do you not feel there is sometimes virtue in exploring the question of psychosocial causation of illness?

Dr. Danes: In my experience, it has led to nothing but disaster. I myself had become so conditioned by psychiatrists' attitudes to the commonness of psychosomatic illness that when I myself fell ill and went to doctors who didn't help me...

Question: When was that?

Dr. Danes: This summer. I went to several physicians who prescribed antibiotics, and I got no better. And the third doctor—I was running a perpetual temperature of a hundred—asked, "Why do you take your temperature every day?" I thought: "Oh well, why on earth *do* I keep on taking my temperature? It must be all psychosomatic, because of the stress of Heather's illness!" I resolved to overcome the problem by sheer brain power—will power. Then a friend insisted that I see a fourth doctor who diagnosed cancer. So I wasn't psychosomatic after all...

Dr. Danes died of mediastinal lymphoma four months after this interview. She had determined, however, to tape it before the disease prevented her from speaking because she wanted others to know of Heather's and her own trials. Her apprehension about Heather's future was based mainly on her fear that her illness would be mismanaged, for Heather is constantly in and out of hospital as her health dictates, a state of affairs that the medical profession refers to as "the revolving door."

Now whenever Heather's malnutrition becomes acute, she is hospitalized to receive psychotherapy and to regain some weight. On one emergency occasion, Heather needed hospital treatment but was out of range of her regular psychiatrist. An internist was pressed into service, and declared, after examining her, that she was receiving far too little medication. With the increased dosage of antipsychotic he prescribed, she was out of hospital in a week, instead of her usual three month stay. Although she obviously had not achieved her ideal weight, she was eating without protest.

However, when she returned to her community care team her dosage was once more reduced and she was back in the "revolving door."

Anorexia nervosa is one of the most difficult diseases to treat. The dysperception suffered by these patients seems to grow worse as the patient becomes thinner; therefore, in order to make any progress in restoring the patient's natural perception and appetite, she (they are mostly women, as it turns out) must first be brought to ideal weight. A vicious circle! Some psychiatrists feel that this process is greatly helped by copious use of major tranquilizers; others disagree. Whether the latter use adequate amounts of medication is not clear. In any event, anorexia nervosa, like other mental illnesses, requires individualized treatment. For Heather, the large doses of major tranquilizers overcame her phobia against food and she gained weight rapidly. It is unfortunate that her community care team, like so many other psychiatric workers, was not alert to incidental findings of helpful therapy, and did not follow through on the cause of her improvement when she left their care for a little while.

In her interview, Dr. Danes spoke of the attempts to drive a wedge between herself and her daughter, and this appeared to be coupled with an attempt to lay the blame for her daughter's illness upon her. There are many other instances of this happening to parents. The mother of a thirty-two year old chronic schizophrenic tells a similar story. Her son had been ill for eighteen years, but was at last being transferred from the mental institution to a half-way house. The psychiatrist in charge of her son ordered her to stay away except at specific times when she would be given permission by a social worker. "We are trying," he said, "to erase your image from his mind in order to create independence." Broken-hearted, she asked, "Why should the image of the one person who continues to love him, whether he's sick or well, be erased from his mind? He will feel I've abandoned him if he can't come home to visit and I can't come to see him! It's such a dreary place that he gets very depressed there!"

Dr. Danes' frustration with the psychiatrist who dismissed her reply with "words, words, words!" has been echoed by many parents who have entered into therapy sessions in a sincere desire to help their ailing children. This refusal to accept words reflects the current nonverbal therapy fad. Our case studies include examples of "face-pushing" to express antagonism, "bopping" to generate anger, speaking "gibberish" to release inhibitions, and nonmusical chairs to delineate family loyalties. There is a case of a patient who refused to return to his therapy group because he could not comprehend how it would help his depression to dredge up anger that he was supposed to feel against his mother who had been dead for twenty years.

Dr. Danes had a healthy response to an attempt to "solicit" her as a patient. She was annoyed and incredulous and turned down the invitation to come into the mental hospital where her daughter was a patient, just as Ms. Smith (see Chapter 10) had done. The trust, constancy, loyalty, and concern that Ms. Danes had for Heather when she was ill are eternal values, but were seen as family pathology by a psychiatrist who wished to evoke anger between mother and daughter. His expectations of this woman reflected a reliance on blind dogma rather than any real acuteness in his sensitivity or his powers of observation.

The contrary view was expressed by Dr. Keith Yonge at a World Federation for Mental Health Meeting when, in speaking of similar matters, he asked whether psychiatrists have forgotten the value of "love, duty, and sacrifice."

When Dr. Danes was dying, Heather in her turn was supportive and loving, demonstrating a strong mother–daughter relationship. Many mothers and daughters who are more suggestible and whose relationship is less firm do, however, suffer permanent alienation.

In contrast to many psychiatrists' attitudes that parents and families are the enemy, it is often found that a patient's adjustment and ability to remain out of hospital is strongly correlated with the presence of a close friend or relative who gives support and sees that the patient takes prescribed medication.

Drs. M. Beiser and L. Jilek-Ali[2] hypothesize somewhat fancifully the opposition as an East–West dichotomy between theories requiring the help and support of the family in treating illness and those we have described. "Most Western psychiatric theories stress the value to the individual of emancipating himself from his family. Asian theories suggest that people must learn to live in harmony with their families and with the past." For some individuals emancipation may be valuable, but during a severe illness, such as cancer, multiple sclerosis, or serious mental illness, it is unrealistic, and may be lethal as well.

Dr. Danes, who died of "psychosomatic" cancer, is entitled to the last word. She wryly compared the modern reliance on the diagnosis "psychosomatic" with Hippocrates' remarks on epilepsy,[3] then called "The Sacred Disease":

> ...it appears to me to be nowise more divine nor more sacred than other diseases, but has a natural cause from

> which it originates like other affections. Men regard its nature and cause as divine from ignorance and wonder, because it is not at all like to other diseases. And this notion of its divinity is kept up by their inability to comprehend it...

Dr. Danes' dying wish to me was that someone write a book on psychosomatic medicine entitled "The New Sacred Disease."

14

Suicide

The case history we shall discuss here was the subject of a considerable amount of newspaper publicity and an inquest at the time it occurred. The material available is therefore considerably more copious and complex than is that in most of the previous histories. In order to treat it as accurately and comprehensibly as possible without risking undue length, we will at times summarize some of the inquest material and at other times quote directly. The complete transcripts of the inquests, as well as our interviews, are, of course available to any student who has a serious interest in the case. We follow our usual practice of changing names and places.

Sara Bowdoin was the third child in a family of four. At the time of the events here described, the twins Deb and Terri, were sixteen, Sara was fourteen, and Cecille was eleven. Their father, Jacques, was a divisional foreman in a large plant; their mother, Annette, was a bookkeeper. They lived in a one-family house in the suburbs.

One Sunday in March, at approximately 8:30 PM, Sara Bowdoin, aged 14, took her life by jumping from a freeway overpass. Only hours earlier she had been discharged from a nearby Mental Health Center after a seven day stay.

The events that led up to her death were uncovered at an inquest, at which the first witness called was Police Corporal John Payne. Corporal Payne described, in dramatic detail, an arduous session that had occurred some weeks earlier during which he had talked Sara down from a position on the railing of an overpass 45 feet above a freeway from which she obviously had intended to jump. With help from the fire department, he succeeded in catching her as she fled, and arranged for her admission to the local general hospital. Corporal Payne's experience left him with the definite impression that this was a serious suicide attampt.

At the time of this first attempt Sara admitted that she had taken 25 aspirin, was given an emetic, and held for observation for a day. Further examination by Dr. Vivien Kent revealed that Sara's physical state was satisfactory, but psychiatric examination was advised and obtained from Dr. Alan Bond, who found her to be "grossly ill and in need of hospitalization" and she was promptly admitted to the Mental Health Center.

The psychiatrist on call at the Center interviewed Sara personally and took a telephone report from Dr. Bond, who noted that she was having visual and perhaps auditory hallucinations, that she was confused, and potentially suicidal. Twelve hours after her suicide attempt, during the interview at the Center, she was no longer confused or hallucinating, but suffered only some residual effects from the aspirin overdose, namely a ringing in her ears and some abdominal discomfort. The diagnosis was reported as "acute brain syndrome from an overdose of aspirin."

The next morning, Dr. Donald Beckman, head of the children's mental health team, read the report and decided that he could not act as primary therapist for the new patient because it would interfere with his treatment of another seriously ill patient. He therefore assigned, as primary therapist, Ms. Josephine Hutchins, who had a Master's degree in nursing and had taken special training in suicide. Ms. Hutchins saw Sara for about an hour a day, either alone or with other nurses, and reported on her progress to Dr. Beckman until the very day she was released, and died.

At the inquest a good deal of time was spent on testimony

reviewing the important problems of diagnosis and treatment. With respect to their decision not to use medication for Sara, Dr. Beckman testified:

> *Beckman:* One of the points we considered was whether medication was necessary for Sara... because some people who are depressed—especially manic–depressive patients, or psychotic depressed patients don't improve, generally, unless they receive medication.... So we were looking to rule out the possibility that she was a manic–depressive. We also wanted to rule out the possibility that she could be schizophrenic... though... she did not have any signs of schizophrenia. She did have some psychotic symptoms prior to coming into hospital... but they were not evident when she came in, and appeared to be related to the overdose of medication. Aspirin in itself can cause hallucinations, as well as confusion and ringing in the ears, which is one of the symptoms that remained when we saw her.

There followed a considerable amount of dispute about whether aspirin could cause hallucinations. Dr. Kent had earlier testified that an overdose of aspirin could cause hyperventilation, flushed face, and agitation and, moreover, could proceed to coma. When asked directly whether hallucinations could result, she replied, "Not as far as I am aware."

Gail Burford, a pharmacist at the government Poison Information Center and lecturer in the Faculty of Pharmacy took the stand. She testified, in part:

> *Burford:* The common symptoms depend on the severity of the overdose... Gastric upsets, later, a little bit of dizziness, ringing in the ears... these may be classified as moderate or severe according to the level of salicylism [aspirin is a salicylate] in the body...
> *Question:* Are you aware of any case where an overdose of aspirin has caused hallucinations?
> *Burford:* Not in my experience, no.

Question: Would it be a rare occurence, in your view?
Burford: It would be an extremely rare occurence.

Ms. Burford then suggested that when Susan had claimed to have hallucinations, tests should have been made for the presence of the types of drugs that were much more likely to be responsible for such manifestations. To a direct question, Burford testified that "Yes, one could expect this type of reaction from one of the hallucinatory type of drugs, the LSD type of drug." [But tests for LSD were not available at that time.]

Dr. Beckman's testimony then continued:

Beckman: So on the Wednesday after I had spoken to Ms. Hutchins, I was satisfied that [Sara] shouldn't have medication for two reasons. One was she didn't show any signs of needing it and the other was to make sure we weren't giving her medication until she was over the results of her overdose.

On the Thursday morning, Ms. Hutchins spent another hour with her, after which she reported to me again that Sara denied having any suicidal intentions. Ms. Hutchins commented that even though Sara denied having suicidal ideas, she knew that she had them, and so questioned her thoroughly about suicide and depression. So it appeared clearly that Sara was not deeply depressed. She was not communicating much about her feelings, but she started to open up, and it appeared that it would be a good idea to have a family meeting the following day. One reason was to obtain more information about Sara's condition and the events that led up to her suicide attempt. Another was to assess the family strengths, and to see how they could be helpful and supportive to Sara. Still another reason was to see what conflicts existed in the family to which Sara might be responding.

Sara did not contribute much to this family evaluation session. Her father testified:

Mr. Bowdoin: I talked to Sara after the session and she said, "Why should I talk to them? When I tell them things, they don't believe me. I tell them I didn't try to commit suicide; they tell me—'We don't believe you! You tried to commit suicide, but you say you didn't know why you were there.'" And that's why she was angry that day.
Dr. Beckman: As a family with some emotional problems, they had some difficulty talking of things which were in conflict.

Dr. Beckman then detailed a number of very common problems, such as a daughter threatening to quit school and another disobeying curfew regulations, all of which, however, had been solved with no great difficulty.

Dr. Beckman: We wanted to find out what effect the family situation was having on Sara. Deb reported that she thought Sara was upset by the conflict in the family...and what we talked about was the fact that it looked as though Sara was the peacemaker in the family, the person who tried to calm things down when there was conflict. And when chores weren't done that would cause arguments at home, Sara would do them, even though they weren't her duty, so that there wouldn't be a conflict. Mr. Bowdoin was able to open up and reach out, and he said that he felt that maybe he hadn't been giving as much love as he could in the family, although he was supplying the material things, he had been a good provider in the family through the years.

Mr. Bowdoin commented later:

"We all felt terrible after the family meetings. We asked ourselves what we were doing wrong. All the little family disagreements were brought out and Sara, you know, she picked up on that. So they decided that she was the sick one in the family because of all our arguments . . . and that therapist suggested that maybe I was giving the family too many material goods and not enough love, and then in court they said that *I* had said that."

In court, Ms. Bowdoin described her daughter:

Ms. Bowdoin: Sara was usually a happy person, especially with my husband. She would joke with him, and if he was in a bad mood because there'd been an argument with one of the children, she would joke with him and try to pull him out of it. They felt that because of this we were putting all our family burdens on Sara's shoulders.

Then Ms. Bowdoin described how Sara would clean house while her mother slept, in order to surprise her, and how she would volunteer to look after her younger sister.

Dr. Beckman continued his testimony at length, basing it primarily on hearsay reports from Ms. Hutchins. He managed to attribute a good deal of professional jargon about cries for help and lifting of burdens from the family to this rather naive fourteen year old girl, and also reported that she was smiling, in a good mood, and evidently possessed with no suicidal ideas. Further:

Beckman: It was pretty clear that the diagnosis was what I call psychoneurotic depression . . . a mild type of emotional illness in which the person is rational . . . the diagnosis appeared quite clear that she was a psychoneurotically depressed girl with some problems with her self image, and with anger against and difficulties with her family.

There was then a good deal of testimony about the reasons for discharging Sara so soon—seven days after admission. The "Health Care" Team asserted that both Sara and the family were anxious for discharge. The family insisted that they had not wanted Sara discharged so soon. Deb confirmed under oath that Sara herself did not wish to be discharged, as did Amy Strange, a girl friend of Sara's who had visited her. In fact, Dr. Beckman admitted that when he raised the question, he thought maybe Sara gave a quiet, "No." The coroner interrupted with his opinion that a "no" was a "no", regardless of its intensity. And although Dr. Beckman testified that he and Ms. Hutchins had arranged for future individual and family sessions, Mr. Bowdoin denies that any specific appointments were ever made.

It was Dr. Beckman's reiterated view that the major factor in Sara's suicide attempt was the "family conflict," and that his opinion had not been changed by her subsequent successful suicide. At this point, one of the lawyers asked why, then, he had felt comfortable in releasing her to her family.

> *Beckman:* Many families have conflicts, especially with teen-agers. It is a difficult time to be a parent—the change from being a child and going on to be an adult—and many families are involved in conflict at that period. This family showed some strength in that they seemed really to care about Sara, and they were reaching out to her. Her sister was close to her and could empathize with her. The parents were willing to come for sessions. So for a number of reasons they had more strength than other families that have conflicts but aren't willing to work them out.

Dr. Robert Wayne, Director of the Mental Health Center, concurred:

> *Dr. Wayne:* Certainly there was disturbance in the family. I don't know of any family in which there is no disturbance at some point during the growth of the children, and particularly in the teenage years. These are very difficult years for the children and for their parents, and particularly in the 1960's and 1970's.
>
> However, we believe that basically the Bowdoin family was a good family, that the parents were loving parents, that they were concerned about their children, that they wished the best for their children...they are basically a healthy family unit that needed assistance in solving a current difficulty...(but)...Sara's difficulties arose in the family...

At this point it might be well to stop for breath. It would appear, on the one hand, that the family dynamics in the

Bowdoin family were sufficiently abnormal and severe to drive Sara to one aborted and one successful suicide attempt, and that she was carrying an intolerable burden as a peacemaker and performer of chores in the family. In addition, although she appeared to be a normal, happy girl with friends both within and without the family, she was diagnosed as a psychoneurotic depressive. On the other hand, we were assured by both Dr. Beckman, who had only two hours contact with the Bowdoin family, and Dr. Wayne, who had none, that all families experience moments of internal conflict, especially with teenagers, and that this family possessed a number of unusual strengths. If the Bowdoin family encountered the same type of conflicts common in families in which there are no suicides, what can possibly be the relevance of an inquiry into those conflicts, an inquisition that Mr. Bowdoin reported had made them all feel terrible? Also, what might be the significance of Dr. Wayne's statement that the 60's and 70's were particularly difficult times to raise children? Perhaps we can deduce the answer from subsequent testimony. A good deal of the cross-examination of Ms. Hutchins had been devoted to the question of streeet drugs, certainly one of the pervasive hazards of the 60's and 70's.

It developed that Sara had been smoking marijuana for an undertermined length of time. As it happens, her school performance had deteriorated during the two years before her death, but Ms. Hutchins had made no connection between this change and the possible onset of drug consumption. Sara had informed Ms. Hutchins that the last time she had smoked was two months before her admission to hospital, and that she did not intend to take up the habit again. When asked whether she had questioned Sara about hallucinations, Hutchins replied:

> Yes, I did. She said at that time that it had only happened on Tuesday night when she had been first admitted, that they were now gone, that the hallucinations consisted of seeing dark shapes that perhaps resembled the face of a

> man, and that is all. She denied having any hallucinations before in her life; she never had that sensation. As for auditory hallucinations, she said that after ingesting the aspirin, she thought she heard music, but that was gone completely. I might add that she was very reluctant to tell me about taking marijuana. She was fearful of her parents finding out and I had to promise to keep any confidences about drugs that she might wish to reveal.

This description of the hallucinations Sara had suffered on the night of her suicide attempt should be compared with a description given by Ms. Hutchins during the inquest.

> *Question:* Did she describe what her trips were like when she had been on marijuana?
> *Hutchins:* Yes, she did. She said she had some trips she found strange, that she had seen some shapes and heard some music, that kind of thing...

The lawyers for the Bowdoins continued to question Ms. Hutchins about Sara's use of drugs and her certainty that she would not smoke again.

> *Hutchins:* The indication was that she had decided on her own, because of other things, such as a good friend of hers who had had a very bad trip on marijuana, that it frightened her, as well as the trip she had, that she didn't like it and didn't want to use it any more.

The nature of Sara's bad trip was never described.

Professor Gil Jamieson of the University Department of psychiatry and an expert on suicide was called to the stand and asked whether a therapist could tell when a teen-aged patient was a habitual user of LSD or marijuana, or when such a patient was likely to return to the use of drugs after release from hospital.

> *Jamieson:* It is difficult to know, because teenagers know that the use of marijuana is frowned upon by most of society. The likelihood of getting honest answers is relatively slim, and, even if you did, the likelihood of them

> telling you how much they smoke and whether they will continue is not very great. So I think you don't have a very great chance of finding out the truth.

When Ms. Hutchins was confronted with this statement, she stated repeatedly:

> *Hutchins:* I have worked with a lot of adolescents and I find that they are pretty straight with me usually . . . I have had the experience with kids that they are usually straight with me . . . In this case, I felt that Sara was being honest with me.
> *Question:* And you routinely rely on those kinds of statements, do you?
> *Hutchins:* Well, I would check it out with other sources.

Ms. Hutchins did not, however, check Sara's statement with other sources before recommending discharge. If she had, she would have found that about a week before her first suicide attempt Sara had attended a pajama party and had been moody, crabby, and different since. "She just wasn't herself, I can't explain," said sister Cecille. Perhaps if Ms. Hutchins had checked these other sources, she might have correlated the uncanny similarity between Sara's hallucinations the night of her first attempt at suicide and the figures she saw and the sounds she heard when she was on a "trip." Furthermore, Ms. Hutchins' insistence on the reliability of her impressions, even after (as we shall see) she knew that Sara had smoked a joint, had perhaps taken a hallucinogenic drug within hours of her discharge from hospital, and had then gone straight to the overpass again can only remind us of the psychiatrist (see Chapter 6) who, virtually over the coffin of a patient who had just killed himself, asserted that the patient wasn't suicidal.

> *Question:* Did you regard the drug use as important?
> *Hutchins:* Not at that time.

After a lengthy interchange on the seriousness with which attempts at suicide by more than one means (drugs and jumping) should be considered, and the importance of soft drug use in the behavior of teenagers, the questioning lawyer finally asked Dr. Beckman:

> *Question:* Did you alter your procedure in your treatment in any way at the Mental Health Center as a result of this incident?
> *Beckman:* No.

We now come to the tragic description of the last hours of Sara Bowdoin, taken from the testimony of her sister, Deb. Early Tuesday afternoon, Sara had been released from hospital and went home with her family.

> *Deb Bowdoin:* We took her home that afternoon, and she was riding the minibike for a while, and then she went inside and started petting the dog, and she was kind of alone at that time. Later on, she and I went down and asked if we could go down to McDonald's. It was about three thirty or four o'clock. So we went down to McDonald's—we took the bus down. We passed the bridge and she was showing me where she was when she tried it the first time. She was showing me where she was, and she didn't look sad.
>
> Well, we came back and went to a friend's house and she offered Sara a joint, and Sara lighted up. That was the only thing in the world she did want, and I said no, but Sara did that and then we went home.
>
> She wanted us to go out later on that night, so we said we were going out. We would meet the others at the gas station around a quarter to seven, and when we got there, we only stayed there for about five minutes. Then we went next door and had a joint between us, but we threw half of it out. So she only had two puffs, and that was two and a half hours before she went up on the bridge.
> *Question:* She was not exhibiting signs of....
> *Deb:* No. She was happy and everything else. She wasn't stoned on two puffs!
>
> Fiona Albert and Amy Strange came about twenty-five after seven, because Fiona owed me some money. I

was supposed to meet her up there. She wanted to talk to Sara behind the gas station. I don't know what about. They stayed there about ten or fifteen minutes talking....After that they came back out, and we stayed there for the rest of the time. About a quarter after eight we were walking home, and we were going to catch a bus after we walked home so that we could go to McDonalds. So we walked home and we got to the bus stop—that's right on Main there—and she said I'm walking down. She wasn't going to catch a bus, she said, and she walked past the bus stop, so we started walking with her. And she stopped and said, "You go ahead of me, I want to be alone. You go ahead of me!" We started walking ahead of her, and we got about half a block ahead of her, and she was still standing there waiting for us to go further on.

Well, we came back and she, I guess she got scared, she crossed the street across Main and she started running down Main on the other side.

We ran after her. Well, before the light, I told her, "Come on, Sara, now stop!" I almost grabbed her but I couldn't, she was running too fast, and she started laughing at that point.

Question: Did she appear to recognize that you were still her sister, that she knew who you were?

Deb: I'm not sure. She ran through the light, the red light. She ran through it—Amy ran through and I stopped at the light. Amy almost got hit running through, so I figured I'd better stop. So Amy went on chasing her, and I caught up to them and Sara ducked into the building and we couldn't find her. When we entered the building she was crossing the street, across Main, so she was heading for the bridge then. By the time she got to the bottom of the bridge there, we were just crossing, and she was up on the bridge, she was just going up.

Question: How far away from you was she then? Half a block?

Deb: About that. She was just on top of the bridge when we were at the bottom. She was about halfway on the bridge and we came toward her and she climbed over and

> said, "Back off!" so we backed off and she came back onto the inside. So we went around to the other half of the bridge and we walked along so we came right directly behind her. I stepped into the middle of the road and she was sort of sitting on the rail saying, "If you take another step I'll jump!"
>
> So I said, "Come on, Sara, we won't tell our parents!" so she said, you know, "Don't take any steps!" So I backed off again, and she goes, "I'll be there in a few minutes." And I said, "How long?" and she said, "A few minutes." And I said, "About five minutes?" and she said, "A few minutes." Then she said, "I just want to think for a while." So she told us to go back to the end of the bridge and wait for her.
>
> So we went back and after about fifteen minutes we were still sitting there and I was going to go and get some help, then I looked over and she was climbing up on the rail. Just then I told Amy, "I'll go call my parents!" and I asked Amy if she'd climbed over and she said "I don't know." So I yelled at her, "Sara, stop!"
>
> And I bent down a little further so I could see between the rails. And that's when she hit the ground.

Where are we now? A fourteen year old girl has committed suicide after brief psychiatric treatment. Is anything to be learned from her history? In retrospect, would a different approach possibly have saved her, or should we accept the view of the Mental Health Center team that Sara's death changed nothing, and that the same treatment methods should continue to be used?

We would like to propose an alternative explanation of Sara's condition, one that might lead to the development of a vastly different treatment regime by a responsible institution, and possibly a different outcome in Sara's case, and no doubt many others as well.

The diagnosis arrived at by the Mental Health Team led by Ms. Hutchins, the primary therapist (see Chapter 8 on the identity crisis in psychiatry), was that Sara suffered from neurotic depression brought about or intensified by family discord. The proposed treatment was "family therapy," which was not very successful because the family could not be gotten together for both family sessions, and because the time allocated to this process was too short. The hallucinations from which Susan suffered at the time of her first attempt at suicide were attributed to an overdose of salicylate.

From our reading of the transcript, and attendance at the inquest, it does not appear that Sara was depressed, either neurotically or psychotically. Whenever her behavior in the Mental Health Center was described, it appeared to be perfectly normal except for some reticence in the early days, understandable enough in a young girl who finds herself for the first time in a mental hospital.

Neither does her behavior at home appear abnormal. She is described as a friendly, cheerful, joking girl. The point, of which much is made by the "team," that she carried a little extra share of the family chores and arguments, would likely be cited as an extra strength had she turned out to be a Florence Nightingale. But, in what we have come to recognize as fairly standard practice in psychotherapy, behavior that would be considered either neutral or laudable in a person who has no problems becomes, mutatis mutandi, sinister pathology once trouble arises.

Sara's presumed neurotic depression was attributed to her role in the family. But when questioned about the safety of releasing her to such a "problem-ridden" family after only seven days, a barrage of testimony from the same team demonstrates clearly that this was a better than average family, and that all families have problems. If all families have problems, why mention them? All families are exposed to the weather, but surely we should not propose that the weather is the cause of such intrafamilial problems as may arise. It appears almost as if the mental health team was willing to tailor its assessment of the family to answer whatever charge it may be confronting at any moment.

To us, the crux of Sara's problem lies in her hallucinations, the observation of strange shadowy shapes, and the hearing of music, which were attributed by the "team" to salicylate intoxication. Since salicylate is a very uncommon cause of hallucination—it is not mentioned as a side effect in Meyler,[1] the pharmacologists' bible on overdose—this diagnosis seems on its face highly unlikely. All testimony at the inquest, save that given by psychiatrists, also denied the possibility. Furthermore, although we do not have reports of Sara's blood salicylate levels available, an approximate calculation can be made from the facts adduced at the inquest. She weighed about 100 pounds and is supposed to have taken about 25 Anacin, a proprietary form of salicylate. A simple calculation of a type that one of us makes every day at work indicates that this would produce a level of about 20 milligrams per milliliter of blood, a therapeutic level that is exceeded frequently in the blood of rheumatics treated with aspirin. That this interpretation is probably correct is shown by the action of the physicians at the General Hospital, who would not have discharged her from observation in a day had she shown a seriously elevated blood salicylate level.

If the aspirin did not cause the hallucinations, what did? Most likely the marijuana she had smoked, or some other hallucinogenic drug. Sara had told Josephine Hutchins that she did not hallucinate when she took marijuana. But when asked, in her language, what her "trips" were like, Sara told her that "... she had some trips she found strange, that she had seen some shapes and heard some music ... " precisely the same phenomena described on the occasion of her suicide attempt.

Ms. Hutchins asserts that her clients do not lie to her and that therefore Sara could not have been taking dope at the time of her suicide attempt. Confidence in one's clients is commendable, but Dr. Jamieson, the Center's expert witness, testified that in such circumstances, "the chance of getting honest answers is relatively slim."

Let us assume, then, that Sara was a perfectly normal girl, who smoked some pot or ate some LSD, like many other teenagers in our psychedelic society, and that the not unusual effect of this indulgence was to make her hallucinatory and suicidal. It is not necessary to infer any state of mental pathology because of her indulgence in drugs; the impression is almost universal that these agents are not harmful, and the matter of use or not is more related to the circles in which a young person travels and to happenstance than to any internal conflict or pathology. But, as was testified by several of the witnesses at the inquest, the use of such drugs can *lead* to serious pathology, including suicide.

What difference would such a view have made to the treatment?

In the first place, the precious few days that were wasted in the painful unearthing of family conflicts that, according to our hypothesis had nothing to do with the tragedy, could have been devoted much more profitably to a serious exploration of the psychedelic drug question. This is also the view taken of the matter by the coroner's jury. After the many hours of testimony and dozens of pages devoted to the exposition of the importance of the family problem and the unimportance of the drug problem by the team, the coroner's jury still brought down the following recommendation:

> We recommend that the Government and the Medical Society consider the establishment of assessment centers to accommodate emotionally disturbed adolescents for a considerable length of time in order that deep seated problems and drug involvement may be uncovered. Such centers should attempt to encourage parents to participate in such treatments.

There was no reason why the Health Care Center could not have served such a role; why they could not have kept Sara for "a considerable length of time," and made whatever effort is possible, with the cooperation of the family, to insure that Sara understood the dangers of her drug taking and to help her fully to realize that she must give up the drugs that had brought her so near to death, drugs which may indeed ultimately have killed her.

Or rather, there was a reason. In our opinion, members of the Health Care Team were intellectual prisoners of the fad of "Family Therapy." In the views they commonly expressed in their testimony, the reason for Sara's problems was the family dynamic, a dynamic that at other times they found to be above average in quality. With such a preconceived notion, it is possible to believe that aspirin causes the same hallucinations as marijuana, that doing a few extra dishes drives a child to suicide, and that parents should not be informed that their suicidal children are taking dope.

Let us return to the Mental Health Center Team's diagnosis of "psychoneurotic depression" to see how this diagnosis and its treatment would be viewed by modern scientific psychiatrists. Donald F. Kline, consultant for the American Psychiatric Association's Diagnostic and Statistical Manual states,[4] "The term 'neurotic depression' is imprecise and obsolete. Therefore, it is not included in the current draft of DSM-III." However, there is a considerable literature making use of this term, and we should give them the benefit of the doubt by seeing whether the "team" made the best use of this literature in their treatment of Sara.

On the evidence, they seem to feel that this diagnosis implies a low risk of suicide, and therefore justifies their early discharge of Sara with no warning to the parents of her suicidal risk. A study carried out by members of the University of Rochester Department of Psychiatry on 179 consecutive suicides[5] found that 25% of the sample consisted of neurotics, "most of them neurotic depressives," whereas the affective psychoses (including psychotic depression) accounted for only 12% of the suicides. A study performed at about the same time in Shropshire, England,[6] showed that "... it is of interest that diagnosis did not give any really worthwhile clues as to which patients might kill themselves." What both studies agree on is that a worthwhile clue is the history of past suicide attempts. They also find that the time of greatest risk is closely related to periods when psychiatric help has been given.[7] In addition, these two studies, as well as one on 100 consecutive suicides by Barraclough[8] and his colleagues, make a point that few of their depressed suicides were receiving adequate antidepressant medication at the time of their successful attempts.

Is the latter finding pertinent in the Bowdoin case? We are assured by Dr. Beckman that his diagnosis of "psychoneurotic depression" precludes any expected benefit from drugs. How does this stand up to the literature?

As long ago as 1961, William Sargant, the dean of writers on physical treatment of mental illness, proposed that MAO inhibitors such as Parnate were of value in the treatment of "atypical" depressives, another obsolete and imprecise category, but one that overlaps the category of neurotic depressive. A study of the effectiveness of MAO inhibitors by Quitkin and his colleagues[9] from that time to the present demonstrates that the MAO inhibitor, phenelzine, "is clearly effective in neurotic or atypical depressives."

So it would appear that even on the basis of their own diagnosis, the mental health center team did not consider Sara's suicide attempt in its true seriousness, and were not aware of the utility of drugs in treatment. Again, we can only suggest in mitigation of their behavior that their adherence to the family causation and therapy system made them feel that they had the situation well under control, and that it was not necessary to be familiar with alternative theses.

The "therapy" inflicted on the Bowdoin family gave rise to a type of pain and suffering that has been written about by James Wechsler,[2] Louise Wilson,[3] and others. Dr. Wayne, in a letter to the medical disciplinary committee, stated, "It is regrettable that the Bowdoin family is burdened by feelings of guilt, in relation to Sara's suicide, but it is impossible for me to see how it would be otherwise." No great perspicuity is required to imagine that it could be otherwise if, first of all, Sara had not committed suicide, and secondly, if the "therapy" had been directed at building up family strengths rather than emphasizing probably non-existent weaknesses.

How do the Bowdoin's feel about the intervention of the Health Care Team? They have expressed their feelings in a letter to the same disciplinary committee, from which we quote in part:

> Although, we understand, there are antidepressants available as treatment for feelings of suicide, our daughter received no medication whatever in hospital and was discharged without medication within a week of admission...
>
> The tone of the session strongly intimated that Sara illness was the result of poor family relations, although Sara repeatedly stated that there was no problem at home or at school. ...The allegations made during the group sessions caused the family an extra burden of pain and self-blame in our grief...
>
> We would also like to have some assurance that other families will not be subjected to similar treatment in the future.

Regardless of the merits of the type of family therapy that is commonly practiced—that is, the attempt to search out causes for serious psychopathology in family dynamics (and we have shown in Chapter 11 that there is no scientific evidence for the validity of this hypothesis), there is no doubt that it regularly causes severe and perhaps irrevocable pain among the family members subjected to it. The alternate approach that we have suggested might not have saved Sara's life. It would, however, almost certainly have prevented the torment of needless guilt and doubt that the Bowdoin family still suffers from. Try as they may, they cannot rid themselves of the thought implanted at two casual family sessions that Sara's illness and suicide may have been caused by the role she was allowed to assume in the family.

15

Warning: May Be Harmful or Fatal If Swallowed

First, do no harm.
—Hippocrates

The caption we have here adopted as our chapter title may be seen on many bottles or cans containing wood alcohol, paints and thinners, insecticides, and other noxious substances that are extremely useful in their proper applications, but should never be ingested. It is becoming increasingly clear, as I hope our chronicles allow the reader to infer, that psychological and psychotherapeutic manipulation may be equally as harmful to the spirit as such physical or chemical toxins are to the body. In the preface of *Evaluation of Psychological Therapies,*[1] R. L. Spitzer cogently remarks that

> For several decades, society has had laws requiring manufacturers of drugs to offer data proving the safety and efficacy of their products before they can be used in treating patients. For a host of reasons, society is apparently unable and/or unwilling to make similar demands of practitioners and proponents of psychological therapies. In the absence of legal requirements, the responsibility of demonstrating the value of the psychological therapies falls to the mental health professions.

We plan here to demonstrate the harmful effects of various "psychotherapies" and to suggest how the public can be warned against swallowing them innocently and without "informed consent."

Just as the contents of some bottles are innocuous or even beneficial, some methods of providing psychological support are to be encouraged. We have already seen how the Clarke Institute assists their patients to live with their disease, brings outpatients together to discuss the side effects of drugs, enlists family aid in management, and generally approaches mental disease in the humane, interdisciplinary fashion we feel is essential to management. Regrettably, their program is a very small exception to the rule of aggressive encounter, provocative therapy, gestalt therapy, est, sensitivity training, and other unproved and likely harmful "psychotherapies."

We have seen many examples in this book where the use of such therapies has led patients to loss of self esteem, to frustration, hospital admission, and attempted suicide, and, finally, to successful suicide, thus justifying the "harmful or fatal" cautionary label we would apply to them. Similar disorientation and suffering are also far too often inflicted upon parents, spouses, and siblings. Are these experiences truly exceptional or are they in fact supported by the literature on the subject?

In the first place, we must reiterate the unhappy conclusion from previous chapters that the amount of research published on the adverse effects of psychotherapy is small. An article entitiled *Contemporary Views of Negative Effects of Psychotherapy*[2] summarizes the opinions of about 100 prominent researchers and practitioners of psychotherapy. The authors state that

> The list of factors that may conduce to negative effects in psychotherapy was lengthy. Deficiencies in assessment were described by many as one of the most fundamental contributory factors, leading to a variety of problems stemming from a failure to identify borderline patients and others for whom psychotherapy may pose serious risks. At a minimum, the misuse of interpretation may promote an unhealthy balance in the patient's life,

> diverting his energies onto the pursuit of insight as an end in and of itself. At its worst, the misuse of interpretation and faulty efforts to produce "insight" may be patently destructive of the patient's psychological wellbeing.

R. L. Spitzer comments that, "Negative effects in long-term out-patient psychotherapy are extremely common." Many of the respondents to the questionnaire of the authors of *Negative Effects of Psychotherapy* commented that psychotherapy often substituted jargon and therapeutic techniques for normal living, reinforcing passivity in the patient's life. Appelbaum said, "Therapeutic work begins to assume priority over other tasks and goals . . . being a good patient comes to assume a higher priority than that of living life to the fullest." Salzman expressed the belief that excessive participation in some of the more radical therapies encourages belief in the irrational as a comfort.

The authors summarize:

> It is clear that negative effects of psychotherapy are overwhelmingly regarded by experts in the field as a significant problem requiring the attention and concern of practitioners and researchers alike.

This widespread concern had already culminated six years earlier in a Task Force Report of the American Psychiatric Association[3] on Encounter Groups and Psychotherapy. This semi-official document refers to group therapy as

> a field notoriously deficient in any systematic research . . . the group offers a unique socially sanctioned opportunity for regressive behavior and impulsive expression. . . . Much more is written about encounter groups than is known about them . . . screening is cursory or nonexistent . . . . Participation should, of course, be voluntary; not only must consent be obtained but *informed* consent. . . . At times the deviant member must be supported in his decision to leave a group which is noxious to him rather than have his free choice blocked by the power of group

> pressure which may threaten, ridicule, or humiliate him into staying.
>
> The intensive group experience is intrinsically neither good nor bad. In irresponsible hands it may result in a host of adverse consequences.... The time is propitious for a research investigation into these issues...

Although the Task Force is alert both to the possibility and occurrence of a "host of adverse consequences," and although they decry the abysmal deficiency of research in the field, they are still prepared to admit that the "intensive group experience is intrinsically neither good nor bad." This is indeed an unusual position to take when one is dealing with a "good" that is marketed at high prices and is widely offered as beneficial for a variety of conditions. The merchandisers of any other product for which similar claims were made would be required to submit thousands of pages of exhaustive research to the FDA to demonstrate that the harmful side effects were negligible, and to the Federal Trade Commission or a similar consumer protection agency to document that the benefit or efficacy was as claimed. In our view, there is already a sufficient literature documenting the harmful side effects of many of these psychotherapeutic treatment schemes that it is questionable whether the FDA or FTC would even accept a brief attempting to show that such side effects are either trivial or nonexistent.

There are a few published reports of research on the long term effects of psychotherapy. Dr. Joan McCord[4] reports on a *preventive* program of psychotherapy started in 1939 on 500 difficult and average youngsters aged 5–13 in Cambridge, Massachusetts. The population was divided at random into approximately equal groups that did and did not receive therapy (counselling). After locating and assessing 80% of the population 30 years later, Dr. McCord remarks ruefully, "The study provides a basis for doubting some of the more basic assumptions—assumptions which I shared—about therapy."

The "solid" negative correlation showed that not only were more men in the therapy group than the nontherapy group convicted of one or more crimes, but that the incidence of conviction increased with time of exposure to counselling, early starting, or with close ties with counsellors. "The results indicate," Dr. McCord devastatingly concludes, "that the most widely held beliefs about therapy may be untenable."

Perhaps these generalizations would be more comprehensible if illustrated by personal experience.

When I was a doctoral candidate in adult education, I attended a two and a half day encounter session directed by a visiting lecturer from the Esalen Institute. Dr. Maupin, in jeans and mod boots, was a swinging young teacher and he mesmerized the highly suggestible group of graduate students, professors, and "people helpers" in his class.

"Walk around the room and hug one another! Everybody hug each other!" he told us, and we did. The class then followed his command to meditate; Dr. Maupin disappeared for an hour's respite. Since I cannot meditate on command, I emulated him and went home and watered my greenhouse plants. When I tiptoed back an hour later, the class was being told to lead our barefoot and blindfolded partners out on the grass to learn trust. (Trusting our partners to avoid the deep precipice to the ocean, or the calling cards of yesterday's dogs?)

When we returned to the classroom, we were told to walk around the room, fully clothed, and look at each other's genital areas. I opted out of that one, but stretched out on the floor for the next exercise.

"Now close your eyes, relax, drop your mind to your chest cavity, your stomach, your pelvic region—now that's a magic region!" Dr. Maupin's voice was enthusiastic. "Savor that region!" he urged. I was willing, but my modest knowledge of anatomy did not allow the fantasy to proceed with any precision.

I might well have fallen asleep, but Dr. Maupin was not through with us. He told us to choose that member of the group to whom we as a group could least relate, and I was then able to observe the vulnerability of the member who had been chosen. Beforehand, he had been outspoken and buoyant with an air of security, and when we had earlier been asked, each in turn, to tell the group why we were sad, he had not, as most of us, blurted out any family problems or personal sorrows. Thus, in the process of ventilating their feelings about him, the objective of the group became to cut this secure and strong-willed man down to size for not "opening up." Harry Stack Sullivan's[5] description of this process is: "If I am molehill then, by God there shall be no mountains!"

In the end, the chosen victim broke down under the group's rejection of him and weepingly related to them an event that might be acceptable as a weakness, specifically that he had had an exceedingly painful leg amputation, but had taken it in his stride and continued his immersion in work and play with his usual optimism, which the group resented. At this confession of imperfection, members of the group hugged him, murmured approval, and accepted him into the society of molehills.

Another attractive, self-assured woman, who maintained her strength through the probings and humiliations of another group, said "I apparently have to show you my broken wing to receive love, and I am not going to do that."

I am afraid that Dr. Maupin did not find me one of the winners in his course. Other members of the group, gushing with enthusiasm, could scarcely wait to tell him how "mind-expanding" the exercises had been. But since I have always felt that it takes months and years to assess another human being, I had refused to follow the leader and had not helped to choose or humiliate the victim. I simply cannot escape the feeling that the adoption of instant human likes, dislikes, and perhaps especially the deeper loving and scorning relationships encouraged by these pseudotherapies, is simply another way to avoid a serious, rational attitude toward people and their problems, an attitude that regrettably seems under harsh attack by so many proponents of the recent fads in the "human potential movement."

When I told an internationally famous physicist at Cambridge University that people in North America often got together for two or three days at a time to spend fifteen hours a day in such groups, his question was, "What business are they transacting? Are they trying to stop nuclear armament, solve the genetic recombination problem, or perhaps come to grips with the energy crisis?" When told there was no objective problem to consider, but simply exploration of the participants' psyches, he was completely incredulous and believed I was putting him on.

I believe that the reaction of Dr. Maupin's sacrificial victim that day helps to explain what happens to any intensely private person who enters hospital in a profound depression, and who suddenly finds that "openness" is mandatory in groups sessions if one is to be allowed to remain in hospital. As one sensitive patient put it,

> Such is the effect of repeated exposure to a certain kind of laughter, that you no longer register what you see, remember what you have learned, or draw fearlessly on what you know to be true. My already low self-esteem was further debased, my loyalty to my family was seen as a sign of craziness, and my depression deepened. Everything that I considered to be a strength or virtue was attacked, and it is only because of my long devotion to these principles of loyalty and truth that I left hospital with some of my old personality and not as an empty shell reconstructed in the image of the group leader.

In similar vein, one of the patients in *The Cuckoo's Nest Revisited* left a group with the remark, "You're really depressing me. I'll go down and slash my wrists."

In 1963, Stanley Milgram conducted an experiment that was, in effect, a test of mindless obedience to authority.[6] Half of his subjects were instructed to press a button that would give shocks up to four hundred and fifty volts to the other half in a simulated behavior modification situation. In fact, there was no power connected to the buttons, but his subjects were not aware of this. To his surprise and the surprise of the world of psychology, he found that fully two-thirds of his subjects pressed the button even when they thought it might injure or kill their opposite number. Milgram's experiment demonstrated that most people are capable of mindless obedience to those in authority.

In a sense, the "people helpers" who were prepared to follow Farrelly's (see Chapter 8) outrageous "provocative therapy" suggestions were pressing the button in the same mindless way as Milgram's subjects. As we are warned in a study entitled[7] *Confrontation: Those Who Qualify and Those Who Do Not,* the process is often used to "vent irresponsible and infantile helper impulses."

When Bill Schutz, the author of *Joy,*[8] told a group of mental health professionals to jump up and down and to yell before he began his lecture to them, the staid professors of psychiatry as well as the psychiatric aides and social workers jumped on command. Such is the power of peer group pressure reacting to the commands of a recognized leader that the embarrassed and flushed professors of psychiatry removed their pipes from their mouths to yell and leap. How can a mental patient undergoing semi-imprisonment be expected to resist the commands of a group leader, whether they are reasonable, or nonsensical and "psychonoxious"?

As though the abuse meted out to patients and their families by psychiatrists were not sufficiently painful, we have shown that a new trend is developing: the partial abdication of medical responsibilities to social workers, psychologists, nurses, and other paramedical members of the community team. A simple example is Ms. Crombie's encounter with the social worker who was perfectly willing and rash enough to misdiagnose her son's problem over the telephone.

In the Bowdoin case (Chapter 14) the primary therapist was the nurse who had initiated confrontative psychotherapeutic approaches with Sara. A study of *Encounter Groups and Other Panaceas*[9] warns that such approaches may pose serious risks for borderline cases.

Perhaps the training received by nonmedical team members deserves as careful scrutiny as that received by psychiatrists. With great sincerity, but little of the scientific knowledge so necessary for making medical judgments, a significant number of social workers and psychiatric aides read the current literature on primal scream, nonverbal techniques, transactional analysis, psychic surgery, fantasy trips, fight therapy, and other courses in the smorgasbord of irrational therapy, and apply them haphazardly. They know that Fritz Perls has said that "the intellect is the whore of the intelligence," and that Gestalt Therapy in which the therapist can tell the patient that she is a "manipulative bitch" is where personality changing is at. In contrast, a brief survey in a city of one million revealed that there were only two library copies of the APA Task Force Report on *Encounter Groups and Psychiatry*. The copy in the medical school library had been checked out twice in nine years, whereas the school of social work copy had been signed out six times. The city's hospital, which requires patients to participate in group therapy, has no copy.

In 1978, Dr. Jonas Robitscher, a lawyer-psychiatrist in Atlanta, Georgia, strongly warned of the growing power of psychologists, nurses, and counsellors. Other research shows that the danger from these nonmedically trained people using random selections from the lexicon of the more than one hundred and forty unproved psychotherapies is very great. Their lack of sensitivity, combined with their confidence in being "up front" is shown (Chapter 11) in the brutal confrontation Ms. Williams suffered at the hands of the social worker who told her she was the cause of her daughter's illness. Ms. Williams is a strong woman, yet she felt humiliated and demeaned by this unfeeling display of hostility. What even more serious suffering might have been inflicted on a timid, worried mother?

There was a time when social workers dealing with mental patients felt that their role was to be nurturing and helpful, to find them homes, jobs, recreation, and friends. Now, as they infiltrate the field of psychiatry, there has been a role change; many of them have become fledgling psychiatrists. They discovered that the encounter movement gave them carte blanche to express their hostile feelings and aggressiveness against their captive audience[10]—mental patients and their families—and thus unwittingly to aggrandize their personal and professional power.

In a study on *Structured Interaction,*[11] Kaplan and Sadock describe their groups. "The therapist chooses a member to be the focus of group activity in a particular session. This technique insures that each member participates and no one withdraws." A patient is thus "up for discussion." The withdrawn or schizoid patient is forced to participate. The authors go on to say that

> "requiring all patients to be discussed in rotation is especially valuable to the schizoid patient. It is unlikely that a withdrawn schizoid patient who is generally difficult to relate to will offer himself up for discussion. He often needs to be selected . . .
>
> The therapist addresses a series of emotionally provocative words or phrases to a patient to stimulate emotional reactions. The purpose of this approach is to encourage communication. Among the categories are: who in the group is ugliest? Prettiest? Least intelligent? Most intelligent? Most sexually attractive? The varieties of categories are endless. Most patients find categories

> anxiety provoking, but they acknowledge that they allow, in fact force one to express feelings that one would never verbalize under normal circumstances.

The reader might see the results of this humiliating experience in Frank's letter (Chapter 1).

In the course of my work, I interviewed a young social worker who was an applicant for a job as a supportive group leader for parents of mental patients. I asked her to tell me about her training in group work. She related that her field placement for the social work degree she was seeking had been at the patient assessment unit in a psychiatric teaching hospital. There she worked under a member of the School of Social Work who had received additional training at "Burning Hills," a local offshoot of the California Esalen Institute. "She was a very confrontative person," said the young applicant. In the group that she had worked with were depressives and schizophrenics. This faculty member had explained her attitude toward these suffering patients to the applicant's class: "We do not allow them to just sit there and observe. They must be made to participate, and if you put them into groups they'll be forced to move!"

One patient had attended the group for three sessions, but had refused to talk. "But then," said the applicant, "the group really got at him at the next session. So after that he reluctantly began to share his dream, which we interpreted as aggression against his parents."

One wonders whether the dream was produced by suggestion or whether, indeed, it was made up from whole cloth by the patient in order to gain approval, just as Eric (Chapter 3) made up dreams when his turn came to "show and tell." We must also remember that there are rare cases of severely ill mental patients who show their aggression against their parents with the business end of a shotgun. This type of suggestion has led Henry Baruk, Chief Psychiatrist at the famous French Hospital at Charenton to say[12]:

> I resent above all the fact that psychoanalysis takes its inspiration from the idea of finding a scapegoat, of encouraging a patient to accuse those around him, his intimates, a situation which creates fresh conflicts among those near to him and often disrupts family peace. This has led me to write elsewhere that psychoanalysis is the greatest manufacturer of paranoiacs that the world has ever seen . . . the psychoanalytic method . . . humiliates the patient in order to discover his secrets.

A rose by any other name . . . Any "therapy" that humiliates, that seeks scapegoats, that inspires accusation is subject to the same criticism. As a matter of fact, Dr. Baruk has made a significantly telling point by attributing this type of activity to psychoanalysis rather than detailing the many tens of other methods now providing distinctions without a difference. Toksoz B. Karasu[13] lists the numerous titles of psychotherapies and shows that they are simply variants of three schools—Dynamic (psychoanalytic), Behavioral, and Experiential.

The young woman finished her interview with me by expressing her enthusiasm for primal scream and bioenergetics as means of ventilating anger. "Of course," she said, "I participated in that with stable people who were screened by a Master of Social Work." Apparently it did not occur to this young professional that there must be something wrong with a system that provides screening for students to make sure they possess the strength to survive this ordeal, yet at the same time forces highly vulnerable mental patients to submit to it.

In a study carried out in California[14] it was shown that 9% of normal, screened, voluntary participants in ten different encounter groups suffered "serious damage," and 33% experienced "negative outcome." Thalidomide was removed from the market and millions of dollars in damages were assessed against its manufacturer for a far smaller percentage hazard.

Although it may seem unfair to compare the deformation

caused by thalidomide with the adverse effects of psychotherapy, we must remember that the latter include some suicides, as well as psychological trauma whose magnitude is difficult or impossible to assess.

The low efficiency and danger that appear to be inherent in "psychotherapy" may in fact result from a philosophical misconception on the part of its enthusiasts.

To trace the historical roots of this misconception, we must go back to 1642, when Rene Descartes, a brilliant French philosopher, tried to create a system of the world by introspection. With a simplistic mechanical materialism coming to be accepted as a result of the discoveries of Galileo (and soon to be immortalized by Newton), combined with his own powerful geometrical ability, Descartes was able to generate a mathematical picture of the physical world in terms of his own invention of analytical or Cartesian geometry. In a sense, he made Greek atomism more precise and mathematical. But this simple atomism could not begin to come to terms with the phenomena of mind and soul, which after all should not be described in terms of the position of points in space.

How to solve the dilemma? "Cogito, ergo sum—I think, therefore I am," enunciated Descartes, thereby giving primacy to the mind. But the connection with the material world was still lacking, so Descartes postponed the problem by taking a position of philosophical dualism. Mental phenomena had their own rules and universe, existing and acting independently of the equally independent and self-ruled material universe.

In some ways, it would appear that psychotherapists are following Descartes. Impressed by the infinite variety and wonder of mental phenomena, and still puzzled by our continuing failure to understand completely the physical basis of mind, they attempt to confine mind to its own independent universe. If the mind malfunctions, it must be treated by mental means—psychotherapy, in short.

From this position stem two serious dangers. In the first place, there is little evidence that mental disease can be treated by psychological intervention. As we have shown earlier, it is much more likely that mental phenomema are a function of the brain—a material system—and that "mental" disorders are really manifestations of biochemical or other biological malfunctions of the brain that can be treated only by attempting to correct this biological dysfunction. The problem resembles an effort that was made some years ago to cure "knock" in internal combustion engines. This faulty combustion of fuel and air could have been attacked on the functional level by working on the "knock"—the malfunction—for example, by providing silencers. The true corrective turned out to be adding substances to the fuel or modifying the chemical structure of the fuel to retard combustion so that no final explosion occurred, thereby suppressing the "knock" along with the loss of power that went with it.

The statement above that there is little evidence that mental disorder can be treated by psychological means seems at variance with the common observation that psychological states can be affected by such means. It is clearly possible to irritate someone into stalking out of a room, throwing down a pen, or even striking the provocateur. Equally, it is often possible to cajole one or many people into performing an act desired by the cajoler, even though it may not be advantageous to the cajolee.

But most such provoked acts are brief, possibly impulsive, and with no permanent effect. Psychotherapies can easily have such effects. We have described a patient being provoked into striking a psychiatric nurse who had constantly insisted that the patient was unloved and unlovable. But the problem in treating mental patients is to correct a whole series of maladaptations that prevent the person from living a reasonably normal life. As we have seen, the patient may not arise till 3 P.M., may hallucinate, may misconstrue messages or the external world, is probably unable to hold a job, and may alienate friends and family. Attempts to correct these flaws on the psychic plane end, more frequently than not, in disaster, major or minor, and rarely if ever have a permanent beneficial impact on the patient's life.

The use of the proper medication, based on correct diagnosis, acting on the *brain* and so, indirectly on the mind, may, on the contrary, improve the patient's symptoms to the point of effective rehabilitation or even, as in the case of some manic–depressives treated with lithium, restore normal personality.

There is a second danger in the *inconsistent* application of mind–body dualism. "I think, therefore I am" can easily be stretched to "I think, therefore I limp, or therefore I bleed." thus leading to the excesses of psychosomatic theory. We have read the horror story[15] of a series of children with a disastrous disease of the central nervous system forced to crawl to the school bus, locked up in solitary for months, questioned about their sex habits at age seven—because of this fundamental philosophical flaw in the training of their physicians. Another such case, described in the New Yorker,[16] is that of a young woman suffering from Wilson's disease, an inborn error of metabolism in which an excess of copper deposits in brain, liver, and other organs. Because her first symptoms were mental, she was considered a suitable candidate for mind treatment. She was exposed to group and individual therapy, successfully encouraged to get a divorce, and to be on the safe side, given shock therapy. A neurologist, who saw her after this process had begun, concurred, although the physician who finally made the correct diagnosis stated,

> Carole was in many ways a classic case.... I'll never forget the look of her. She *looked* like Wilson's disease. She had the typical masklike face and the fixed and twisted smile.... I thought Kaiser-Fleischer rings [in the irises] were grossly visible... distinctive slurred speech and that typically squeaky voice.... It was all there. She was practically a textbook presentation. I think my secretaries could have made the diagnosis.

What this young woman needed was penicillamine, a chemical that removes the copper from the vital organs and prevents further deterioration. What she got was psychotherapy, agony, divorce, and additional deterioration of liver and brain while the witch's sabbath played itself out.

The harm resulting from psychotherapy is not restricted to patients. Since many of the psychotherapies consider it axiomatic that mental illness stems from faulty interpersonal relations, they often seek, and, because of the nature of the search and the search process, find, causative problems between the patients and their loved ones. Often a parent may suffer as much as or more than the patient.

Grace, the daughter of Prof. Andrew Bridges, became ill at age fifteen. She lost weight almost to the point of diagnosis of anorexia nervosa, suffered from decreased energy and nervousness. Daughter and parents attended a psychiatrist who repeated to them the Greek myth of the unresolved sexual attraction between father and daughter. To gild the lily, he accused the loving, concerned, gentle mother, who adored her daughter, of competing sexually with her. The splendor of affection Prof. Bridges held for his daughter was disrupted. Never again did they recover their old intimacy until three months before her death from leukemia, five years later. Her father is convinced that her early symptoms owed to her preleukemic state. Perhaps the disease would not have been discovered even if the diversion of the Oedipus Complex had not been raised. But the Bridges would have been spared the agony, suspicion, and self-blame that resulted. "I withdrew when she needed me most," said Prof. Bridges.

Many families have been subjected to separation techniques. In the view of the psychotherapists, the children are dependent upon their families, or under some other baneful family influence. When Doris McPherson's daughter was in hospital, a strenuous effort was made to separate her completely from her family. When the family visited, they were denied a meeting with Jane, until once, when the parents insisted, they were reluctantly allowed to spend a short time with her in the constant presence of a nurse, so that "we were unable to speak to her privately. Jane just cried and held me tight the whole time."

After Jane's suicide, her friend told the family that Jane didn't know why the family were not visiting her; she thought they had forgotten her. The McPhersons were told that Jane did not wish to see them. Was the perpetuation of the deception the reason for not allowing the family to speak with her privately?

These examples of cruel and unusual punishment meted out to families and patients could be multiplied indefinitely. The therapy on which they are based is harmful to some, and fatal to others, who must indeed swallow them for lack of an alternative.

It is probable that psychotherapy, based as it is on a fundamental misconception of nature, cannot provide beneficial results for mental patients. The professional Task Force of the American Psychiatric Association, although aware of the hazards and lack of validation of group psychotherapeutic methods, is not prepared to go so far. They do, however, make clear the experimental nature of the process, and insist that it be performed only on screened volunteers giving *informed* consent, as with other experimental procedures.

In practice, this injunction of the APA is completely disregarded, both in letter and spirit, with respect to mental patients. We have seen mental patients forced to leave hospital if they would not participate in group therapy, and of course staff and fellow patient pressure keep many participating against their will. "Informed" consent is a mockery when the group leaders themselves are often quite uninformed about the hazards of their activities.

Martin Gross[17] points out that some hospitals recognize

that the important treatment for hospitalized mental patients is *medical* treatment.

> At Springfield Hospital, a state institution in a London suburb, patients live in a cheerful, sympathetic atmosphere. They come in desperately ill, and are given the same medical treatments as in American hospitals. They leave greatly improved *without* having received psychological intervention, either in the form of psychotherapy or as extensive probing to find the supposed childhood cause of the illness.... In England, psychotherapy is almost toally divorced from the treatment of the ill.

How does the North American public feel about the enforced exposure to experimental procedures of people unable to make a free choice? In 1968[18] and again in 1979[19] carefully constructed public opinion polls queried a wide variety of citizens about their attitudes toward participation of various groups in experimental medical procedures. That the respondents were not exceptional or overly altruistic is shown by the fact that they volunteered others for the experiments about twice as frequently as they volunteered themselves. But both surveys showed an inordinate unwillingness to allow captive audiences to be used for these purposes. Only 4% of those polled in the 1968 study and 20% in the 1979 study expressed a willingness to allow institutionalized psychiatric patients to be used for medical experiments.

So we find mental hospitals carrying out mandatory, experimental, and hazardous procedures that are condemned both by an overwhelming majority of the North American public and by the American Psychiatric Association. The American Public probably does not know; the Psychiatric Association cannot plead ignorance.

There ought to be a law.

16

Erewhon Revisited, A Psychoparable

And was Jerusalem builded here, among these dark Satanic mills?

—William Blake

In the year 2072, 200 years after Erewhon was visited by Samuel Butler, a delegation from 1980 materialized through the time portal. The party revisiting this famous but mysterious country were, as it happens, particularly interested in the treatment of mental patients. They were welcomed as honored guests and referred to the Minister of Mental Health, Dr. Graham, a gentleman of indeterminate age, with gray hair, a rather erect and athletic bearing, and a presence that was at once humble and arresting. In his modest office, which was ten by fourteen feet and contained a small desk and several simple but very tasteful paintings, was a plaque that announced[1] "Psychiatry is the practice of neurology without physical signs."

After welcoming his guests, Dr. Graham asked what he could do to help them. The spokesman for the delegation explained that the situation back in 1980 was sheer and utter chaos: Mental patients were ill-treated; factions and schools of treatment engaged in internecine warfare; the costs of the chaos were constantly increasing to no benefit; a certain amount of promising research that had already achieved good results was generally ignored, or not being applied to any healing purpose; and that, because of Erewhon's geographical isolation and temporal location in the future, they had come to learn whether some of these problems may have been solved by the Erewhonians. In short, the delegation imagined that the Erewhon experience would be of high value to them when they returned to their own times.

Dr. Graham responded: "Well, I am very happy to have the opportunity to help you with this problem because indeed you are correct. We have solved these problems here, but we have been through periods very much like those you describe.... In fact, I have experienced them myself. As you may know we in Erewhon live a longer and a healthier life than people from outside, and I am older than I appear to be. I can tell you a good deal of the history of the problem from my own experience, and I am also able to discuss what occurred in earlier times because my interest has led me to conduct historical research on the subject.

"Back in the time you inhabit, the situation in Erewhon was not very different from yours. We too had our cults; we too had our gigantic mental insitutions that were something between a prison and a lunatic asylum; we had our "mental health care teams" that were havens, not indeed for the patients, but for the abundance of social workers and psychologists that proliferated at the time, and for many nurses who had no desire nor aptitude to nurse. Our psychiatrists attempted to be psychologists; our psychologists attempted to prescribe medication; the patients were blamed for their illnesses, or if they were not, their parents and families were scapegoated, and there was general agony throughout the community. The medical profession had failed abysmally in the treatment of seriously ill mental patients, and because of this failure, and because of self doubt, they were quite inconsistent in their choice and use of psychiatric methods. Unlike other specialties, whose practitioners intensify their ministrations as the patient's condition worsens, psychiatrists shipped their sickest patients to large institutions where genuine care and help for the patient were almost nonexistent, where in effect the patients were merely incarcerated, and where in most cases, the psychiatrist never saw them again. However, although there was hardly a psychiatrist who did not use medication on mental patients, they had no clear idea of what they were doing. Many of them thought that the medication's sole value was to make the patient more amenable to whichever one of the hundred and forty psychotherapies (proliferated from the three original branches) they desired to explore at the time, rather than as specific pharmacological correctives for various pathologies or deficiencies in the brain chemistry of the patients. Inasmuch as these "hundred and forty psychotherapies" were not medical treatment, in any sense of the word, it became common for nonphysicians to set up as practitioners of their own often parodistic versions, and indeed one can see that there is no reason why a social worker, a psychologist, an ex-nurse, or a psychological aide cannot administer primal scream therapy, sensory deprivation, laying on of hands, striking with styrofoam bats, or any of the multitude of these clearly abusive or nonsense therapies with equal deftness, and probably with no worse result than a medically trained person might. There were at that time many hospitals, many institutions, in which the personnel greatly outnumbered the patients, and in which no effort was made to discover whether the patient was being benefited or indeed harmed by the treatment being administered." Graham then quoted a critic from the visitor's own times, Dr. Henry Miller[2]: "Since the flight into so-called dynamic psychiatry with a speculative and entirely affirmative basis in psychological determinism, psychiatry has suffered from a surfeit of complex and unprovable theory and a dearth of simple testable hypotheses." Dr. Graham continued: "This is what your situation was, and indeed it was deplorable, nor did there appear to be any way out of it. The mentally ill had great need and few advocates, whereas the fad pushers, the psychotherapeutic exploiters had powerful outlets and many evangelists.

"The virus of the theory of the psychological causation of physical as well as mental illness was so widespread that it was adopted not only by psychiatrists, but by general practitioners who, over the coffee table, could be heard telling each other that eighty-five percent of the people who come through the door haven't anything wrong with their bodies, just in their head, with surgeons who felt that duodenal ulcers and ulcerative colitis were essentially psychological diseases, and with neurologists who thought that migraine was caused by stress. And it seemed the psychosomatic theory of mental illness was so firmly entrenched that it would never be dislodged.

"However, a 'small cloud, no larger than a man's hand' was already appearing on the horizon. There were people who, in seeing the chaos, felt that there must be a better way out. These generally were scientifically trained physicians, who recognized that the brain was one of the largest, and by far the most complex and energy-consuming organ in the body. They further recognized that it would be astonishing if this organ did not suffer a range of aberrations as diverse as those the heart, the liver, the lungs, and all the other organs and systems of the body fall prey to. In the belief of the scientific psychiatrists, it was entirely reasonable that disastrous changes in a person's mental outlook, such as rapid fluctuation from a state of such abject depression that the afflicted one is unable to get out of bed directly into a manic state in which that patient moves twice as fast as normal, survives without sleep, and has three hundred ideas per hour, could only arise from some chemical malfunction or physical defect in the brain, and not from some early psychological trauma. By 1990 these people had at last managed to organize at the University of Erewhon a special course, which they called psychoneurology, in which all students were required to have an extensive background in either biological or chemical science before they received the usual common medical training. Following this training they then underwent four years of rigorous education and research in neuroanatomy, neurochemistry, and clinical neurology. Only when this had been completed were they allowed to serve an internship in the still existing mental hospitals.

"When the physcians given this new training came to see seriously ill mental patients, they scrupulously avoided postulating psychological cause or cure for a disease that was obviously biologically based. They were also familiar with the rather sketchy, but interesting scientific literature up to your time demonstrating that many mental and other illnesses leading to psychological manifestations were based on clearly definable biological disorganization. They realized, for example, that people with hyperactivity of the adrenal glands or the thyroid gland could show symptoms indistinguishable from those of ordinary mental patients. They realized that people who had ingested certain toxins such as LSD might have symptoms mimicking mental illness. And so it was a small step to believe that serious mental illness was also chemically and biologically caused. They were familiar with the work of Roger Guillemin, who won the Nobel prize in dimmest 1977 for the isolation of hypothalamic hormones, and of scientists such as Solomon Snyder, Hans Kosterlitz, Candace Pert, and John Hughes, who discovered the brain-secreted "endorphins" that had morphine-like effects both in their ability to decrease pain and to improve a patient's affect and the brain's own opiate receptor. They were familiar with the work of Dr. Horrobin in Montreal, who suggested that schizophrenics suffer from a deficiency of prostaglandin, and that drugs that raise its level, such as penicillin, appeared to ameliorate their condition. They went back further into scientific history and studied the writings of Dr. G. Stanley Hall of Johns Hopkins

University a century earlier. Hall, a giant in the field of adolescence and founder of the Journal of Genetic Psychology, had observed that very often mental breakdowns occurred when what he called the 'sturm and drang' of adolescence wreaked its toll on the sensitive bodies, including the brains, of people whose hormonal balances were changing rapidly.

"In 2017 the psychoneurology lobby succeeded in passing legislation to place all methods of psychological manipulation under the control of the Pure Food and Drug Act. For the first time it had to be proved that a method such as primal scream was 'efficacious for the purpose claimed, and not harmful' before it could be sold to the public,* just as had earlier to be proved for drugs and medical devices. The number of psychotherapies fell drastically.

"The year 2020 produced another landmark. A book called *Emotional Catharsis: squeezing the pus out of your psyche,* was published. Although it passed the board of review of the Pure Food and Drug Commission, a notice was required to be printed in large letters on both book jacket and title page: 'Warning: The Surgeon General states that this treatment may be harmful to your mental health.' This was of course the last book of its kind published.

"When the psychoneurologists were released into the community, even with no better tools for treatment than were available to you in the 1980's, they promptly made vast improvements in the lives of the mental patients and incidentally, and it's not insignificant, vastly decreased the cost

---

*Editor's Note: In 1976, R. L. Spitzer and D. F. Klein wrote in the preface to their book *Evaluation of Psychological Therapies,* Johns Hopkins University Press, pg xiii, "For several decades, society has had laws requiring manufacturers of drugs to offer data proving the safety and the efficacy of their products before they can be used in treating patients. For a host of reasons, society is apparently unable and/or unwilling to make similar demands of practitioners and proponents of psychological therapies. In the absence of legal requirements, the responsibility for demonstrating the value of the psychological therapies falls to the mental health professions."

of treating those patients. They held firmly to the opinion that these people were biologically sick; there were no more disputes about whether mental illness existed; they did not tolerate the quackery and faddery of the 140 psychotherapies. Believing as they did that mental disease was a chemical disease, really a disease of the brain rather than a psychological one, they proceeded to use the medical treatments then available, which were basically the same primitive drugs you had at your disposal in the 1980's: phenothiazine, antidepressants, MAO inhibitors, penicillin, endorphins, and the like, but they used them in a sort of last ditch battle against the disease. First of all, they were careful to diagnose and eliminate any recognizable physical disease, which many of these patients have, and to improve their physical health by diet, by vitamin and mineral supplementation, and by exercise. They then proceeded prudently to employ the psychopharmacologic armamentarium that they believed in and with which their training had made them very skillful. If their treatment did not succeed, the patient was reassessed until they had identified the correct symptom complex or ferreted out the correct diagnosis, and all further treatments attempted to take specific account of the biological individuality of that patient. As you know, one person is often found to require five times as great a dose of a drug as another to realize the same effect. They measured the blood levels of these drugs, they experimented with new drugs, and they found that some 90–95 percent of the patients could be rehabilitated by these means. Indeed they were not cured, they could not be discharged without the drugs, and even when staying carefully on this regimen, they were not restored to their pre-morbid selves, though they generally survived in one fashion or another.

"The molecular neurologists also made a serious effort, which had rarely been attempted earlier, to see that those patients who were released to the community took their medication, that their progress was vigorously followed up, and that the medication was changed as their biological states changed. Just as a diabetic who is perfectly balanced on a certain amount of insulin can suddenly require much more, for example, under the stress of trauma or infection, so a mental patient may require a drastic change in the dosage of balancing drugs to maintain the same state of mental health when physically or psychologically stressed.

"During this transitional period, there were molecular neurologists in some of the key positions, and old-time psychiatrists in some of the others; we had the romantically named Glenhavens, the gigantic post-nineteenth century institutions side by side with the general hospital psychiatric wards, which were miniature versions of the Glenhavens, and the occasional sort of Crazy Hilton attached to a University department of psychiatry. Regrettably, agonies and disasters continued to occur in the institutions that were run on the older lines.

"For example, in the course of my research I ran into a rather pathetic case history of a woman some 65 years of age who had been in the enormous state institution, Glenhaven, for 35 years, and had been doing rather well there. She certainly was not in an inappropriate place because she was seriously ill, but she was reasonably happy, and she managed a few small activities. She did some knitting and she read a little bit of newspaper each day; she was in good physical health. During this transitional period many of the larger insitutions were being shut down or decreased in size, and since she was doing so well, she was chosen as one of the people who should be repatriated to the community. She was sent to a rather dismal boarding house—parenthetically I might remark that in those days the boarding houses were private enterprises not necessarily run by people who were enthusiastic advocates of the mentally ill, nor by people of high sympathies, but rather, who were often running them simply as businesses. But the conditions in the boarding homes were not appreciably worse than they had been in the big institutions. Surprisingly enough, although it was not discovered by the authorities (or perhaps it was not surprising), this woman went into a prompt decline and was utterly depressed for a six month period. She could not rise from her bed, she lost 40 pounds, and was on the verge of death. One of her relatives, after repeated visits and watching her go down hill, made sufficient contact with her to find out that there was indeed a very good reason for this decline. It was this. In her 35 years in Glenhaven she had had as a constant companion another woman who was about the same age, of the same background, and who suffered a very similar sort of illness. The two of them had together constructed a communal fantasy world that protected them from the unpleasantness of their disease and surroundings. When the ward was broken up, no effort was made to determine whether any such friendship patterns existed or whether there were special reasons for moving people either in groups or as individuals. One would have thought that the social workers, of whom there were many in this hospital, would have considered this to be one of their primary responsibilities. But the social workers were busy taking courses in psycho-bopping, primal scream, behavior mod, and assertiveness training, and were experimenting with these therapies on the patients. No one thought to investigate the sociological microcosms that existed, which a social worker presumably is trained to do, and which they had done in previous years, before they became therapists. And so, these two elderly and rigid people, whose only grip on reality was their relationship with each other, were separated and sent to distant boarding houses, and they reacted very badly.

"This happened time and time again, though it is extremely difficult to document. We seem to find this view implicit in most of the private correspondence in our archives, though it was seldom published, because it was not the habit of the psychotherapeutic community of those days to immortalize their failures in the patient histories, if, indeed, they were even remotely aware that they had failed. The lack of peer review in this specialty made the omission all the easier.

"By the year 2030, mental hospitals and psychiatrists had both been abolished, just as had been predicted by psychiatrists in your time. This resolution came about in a rather interesting way, connecting up with the same Dr. Miller to whom I have referred previously. In his humorous fashion he had tried to establish a Society for the Abolition of Psychiatrists during the latter half of the twentieth century. This society did not actually receive a government charter, although some of the applicants for membership came from the ranks of the world's most eminent psychiatrists, as well as from the patient rolls. The Society never came into existence because by that time it was no longer necessary. The psychiatrists had become so involved in fighting battles over putative heresies, in protecting themselves from the inroads of psychologists, social workers, and so on, in hiring peripatetic lecturers to orate on psychotherapeutic deficiencies, that there came a year when no one passed the certification examination. At this time, although it was very much contrary to medical tradition, the certifying body held a meeting and formally disbanded the specialty of psychiatry. Fortunately, of course, there were already a large number of psychoneurologists, and they more than took the unmourned place of the psychiatrists.

"Incidentally, although it was not realized at the time, this profession of psychoneurology was in a sense a cyclical return on a higher level to an earlier period, one in which the psychiatrists themselves had grown out of the ranks of the neurologists and had held titles such as 'neuropsychiatrist'. The inversion of the prefix and the suffix in this title points to the much heavier emphasis on neurology in our time than it did in that period.

"The abolition of the mental institution, the large crazy house, had an even more interesting history. One of the new psychoneurologists, observing the appalling conditions in Glenhaven, the state institution to which he was assigned, and the antitherapeutic effect of the circumstances of enforced incarceration, chronic hospitalization under callous and brutalized staff* (I almost said guards), spent much of his time reading the history and philosophy of mental insitutions. He came upon an official government report† opining that the best thing to do with the very Glenhaven about which he was brooding was to dismantle it brick by brick, accompanied by a ceremonial salute to the end of barbarism. Although he obviously did not have the power to follow this (possibly tongue-in-cheek) advice, the young man was full of resource and energy. He had himself appointed head of a new committee on handling of major emergencies, evoked a nuclear bomb drill in which all patients and staff were evacuated to a distance of five miles, and calmly and methodically burned the institution down. In his usual thorough way, the job was done so that it was impossible to stop the fire and, indeed, it cost only a trivial sum to remove the minor debris that remained. Naturally, this incident caused quite a bit of comment and investigation. In the ensuing publicity, everything I am telling you now came to light, and there was a great deal of sympathy for the act that the young man had undertaken. In fact, the sympathy was so extensive that when he finished serving a very short jail term, he was appointed the head of the new Commission on Mental Health. For the first time the term mental health, to paraphrase Samuel Johnson, was not like the

*Editor's Note: There was a curious and now famous rash of charges, in November, 1976, accusing workers in mental hospitals of choking, strangling, drowning, and murdering up to 1179 patients. For example, see San Francisco Chronicle, Nov. 17, 1976. "Sacramento Investigators have uncovered 36 'very questionable patient deaths' in a probe of 10 state mental hospitals . . . there is a possibility that at least some of them may lead to murder charges." . . . a hospital employee testified that he choked a patient unconscious just before the patient died."

†See *Psychiatry at the Crossroads,* a special report to the Minister of Health of British Columbia by Dr. R. Foulkes, July, 1974, p. 15.

word virtue in the mouth of a whore. It had some true significance because his effort genuinely was to establish mental health, not simply to use the term euphemistically to conceal an uncaring malpractice.

"So we reached a point at which there were no mental hospitals, there were no psychiatrists, but there were still mentally ill people. We had not then, as we have now, solved the problem of mental illness. Then how did we get along?

"In the first place, one might imagine that perhaps even in your time no harm would be done by the abolition of mental institutions and psychiatrists altogether. But we had positive plans as well, and we did manage to get along even better.

"We did not allow the beautiful grounds, which were the only glory of the old Glenhaven Hospital (snakepits always had such idyllic names) to lie fallow or to be developed into suburban sprawl. Very quickly we constructed on this site what at first glance would appear to be a lovely university campus. It contained small residences of various kinds for couples, for small families, or for groups of single individuals; it contained common dining rooms for unsegregated use by the staff and patients, as well as private kitchens; it had workshops for a variety of small industries that varied from very simple to very complex. It incorporated recreational facilities, both athletic and individual; it contained a shop for the execution of artistic programs at which many of the mentally ill have been known from time immemorial to excel.

"It is probably not at all accidental that so many outstanding artists and musicians throughout history have been either borderline or overtly schizophrenic. People such as Van Gogh, Nijinsky, who spent most of his adult years in mental institutions, Schumann, and many others. The painting of a considerable number of late twentieth century artists of extremely high quality exhibits many of the properties shown by the painting of schizophrenics. In any case, an opportunity was afforded for the encouragement of vastly different perceptions, which on the one hand can signify mental illness, and which on the other hand make it possible to portray the world in such graphic terms. Not only was the time of residence on this campus thoroughly planned, so that the patients did not suffer the ennui and feeling of worthlessness that are common in mental institutions, but they were also encouraged to develop a pride in their work and work habits, a welcome desire to awaken in the morning and carry on in the ways in which normal people do.

"There were also quiet places to rest, to contemplate, and to escape from the pressure that so often is associated with an acute attack of these illnesses, just as any other illness, and that leaves the affected individual in no mood to paint paintings or write symphonies,, or even to make brooms or build computers. This emotional shelter is something that generally had not earlier been available, and evokes the statement of your once popular author, Allan Watts, who had said that 'mental patients need an Ashram, not a hospital.

"A modest number of these patients, after some months or years on proper medication, with a healthful regime, working under these genuinely therapeutic circumstances, and developing their egos and bodies, were able to leave the campus and be restored to a normal place in society. Some of them, indeed, became capable of this, but chose nonetheless to remain on the campus. Since the activities provided there were productive and partially self supporting, there was of course no reason why they should not be allowed to stay. Others did not recover quite so readily and lived their lives out peacefully on the campus in a manner that would not have been possible under any other circumstances.

"The point to the whole operation is that there was a truly multipronged attack on an extremely complicated problem, but one that was fundamentally biochemical and medical, that recognized the biological origin and significance of mental disease, but did not stop at medical treatment. Indeed, no rehabilitative medicine can or should stop at medical treatment, because any person chronically incapacitated with a medical or surgical disorder suffers additional problems that other people do not, and requires support from people with all manner of skills, and all manner of sympathies. On the other hand, they do not require a hospital environment after the acute illness is over, a very simple fact that lay at the basis of our rehabilitation program, which has now been proved to work very well, and very economically.

"The sequel to this story is possibly of some small interest to you, though I shall not discuss it in detail. It is that we now see even this system as outmoded. Because of the special understanding our society has brought to the biological basis of mental illness, we have strongly supported fundamental research, and all of the wildly unlikely theories and fads that had so totally failed to address the biological bases of mental disease have shriveled and disappeared. We also recognize that the crucial trial of any new development in research must be carried out under scientific circumstances, and because our psychoneurologists were on the wards as well as in the laboratories, the result was that within fifty years after the abolition of psychiatry, we abolished all mental illnesses, just as you had earlier abolished smallpox. We have now identified all of the biological causes and have found simple physiological treatments that are applied in a humane and supportive framework. These insights have also led us to evolve a social framework that strongly ameliorates the psychological atmosphere that in earlier eras assured a rapid descent into intractability once the physical disease had actually begun to manifest itself.

"Some people still manage to escape the preventive methods that we have set up and become mentally ill nonetheless. This lasts only a short time; they are quickly identified by the general physicians who are now routinely trained in psychoneurology to recognize mental illness, know how to deal with it, and can refer patients for the true cure—not the management, but the cure.

"I will not go into details of the causes and cures for mental illness, because the nature of the time transition mechanism that has brought you here to Erewhon in the year 2072 does not allow such scientific information to be carried back. It will unfortunately be necessary for you to repeat the arduous investigations that we had to carry out, but perhaps it will be somewhat easier for you knowing that the problem is indeed susceptible of solution.

"And you should not be too pessimistic about the time scale that will be required for your change. Already the signs are appearing that the stage is being set for it. In 1979, Dr. Robin M. Murray of the British Institute of Psychiatry, wrote[3] *A Reappraisal of American Psychiatry.* His conclusions were:

> Remarkable changes have taken place in American psychiatry over the past 20 years. The era of psychoanalytical supremacy has passed, and realism is replacing the exaggerated claims which were made of psychiatry's ability to produce personal, social, and even political change. The importance of phenomenology and accurate diagnosis is increasingly recognized, and American researchers have made impressive contributions to psychiatric genetics and psychopharmacology. Despite these advances, office practice generally continues to function on an outmoded model, and psychiatric resources remain inequitably distributed.

"So the abuses and agony-creating therapies which, I know, disturb many of you, are the visible, painful result of cultural lag, of the continued application of theories that are, even in your own time, obsolete. But it is only a matter of time—and it may even be a short time—until the new research and the new teaching penetrate to the level of practice. And when that time comes, you will have reached Erewhon."

Bibliography

Chapter 1

1. Friedmann, Claude T. H., "Psychiatry and Psychotherapy: Is a Divorce Imminent?" *The Western Journal of Medicine,* **129,** no. 2, 156–169 (1978).
2. Editorial, "Parents of Psychotic Children," *British Medical Journal,* 379–380 (18 Nov., 1972).

Chapter 2

1. Zimbardo, Philip, *Shyness: What it is and What to do About It,* Addison Wesley, Reading, Mass. 1977.

Chapter 3

1. Janov, Arthur, *The Primal Scream,* Nichols, Great Britain, 1970.
2. Research Task Force of the National Institute of Mental Health, *Research in the Service of Mental Health.* Julius Segal, Ed., NIMH, Rockville, Md.; DHEW Publication NO (ADM) 75–236, 1975, pg. 324.
3. Ross, Val, "The Great Psychiatric Betrayal," Saturday Night, Toronto, 17–23 (June, 1979).
4. Vonnegut, Mark, *The Eden Express, a personal account of schizophrenia,* Praeger, New York, 1975.
5. Glasser, William, *Reality Therapy,* Harper and Row, New York, 1965.

6. Baruk, Henry, *Patients are People Like Us, the Experiences of Half a Century in Neuropsychiatry,* Morrow, New York, 1978.
7. Torrey, E. Fuller, "The Primal Therapy Trip," *Psychology Today,* 62 (December, 1976).
8. Ibid, p. 64.
9. See ref. 2, p. 324.

Chapter 4

1. Fieve, Ronald R., *Moodswing, the Third Revolution in Psychiatry,* Morrow, New York, 1975.
2. Katz, Sidney, "Lithium for Alcoholics?" *Homemakers,* 68 (May, 1977).
3. Merry, J., and Reynolds, C. M., "Prophylactic Treatment of Alcoholism by Lithium Carbonate," *Lancet,* 481–482 (4 Sept., 1976).
4. See ref. 2, Chapter 3, p. 179.
5. See ref. 13, Chapter 5.
6. Hansen, H. E., and Amdisen, A., "Lithium Intoxication," *Quarterly Journal of Medicine,* New Series XLVII, No. 186, 123–144 (1978).
7. Forrest, John N., Jr., et al., "On the Mechanism of Lithium-Induced Diabetes Insipidus in Man and the Rat," *Journal of Clinical Investigation,* **53,** 1115–1123 (1974).
8. Hestbech, J., et al., "Chronic Renal Lesions Following Long-Term Treatment with Lithium," *Kidney International* **12,** 205–213 (1977).
9. Seeman, Mary V., "Management of the Schizophrenic Patient," C.M.A. *Journal* **120,** 1097–1104 (May 5, 1979).

Chapter 5

1. Committee on Nomenclature and Statistics, American Psychiatric Association. *Diagnostic and Statistical Manual,* draft second edition, third printing (DSM-II), American Psychiatric Association, Washington, 1978.

2. R. J. Stoller, et al., "A symposium: Should Honosexuality Be in the APA Nomenclature?", *American Journal of Psychiatry,* **130,** 1207–1216 (1973).
3. Seymour S. Kety, et al., "Mental Illness in the Biological and Adoptive Families of Adopted Individuals who have become Schizophrenic: A Preliminary Report," In Genetic Research In Psychiatry, R. R. Fieve, et al., ed., Johns Hopkins University Press, Baltimore, 1975, p. 147 ff.
4. S. Kety, et al., "Genetic Relationships within the Scizophrenia Spectrum: Evidence from Adoption Studies," in *Critical Issues in Psychiatric Diagnosis,* R. L. Spitzer and D. F. Klein,eds., Raven, New York, 1978.
5. Gershon, S., et al., "Drugs, Diagnosis, and Disease," in *Biology of the Major Psychoses; A Comparative Analysis,* Daniel X. Freedman, ed., Raven, New York, 1975. p. 91–92.
6. Benedict, Ruth, *Patterns of Culture,* The New American Library of World Literature, New York, 1934.
7. Murphy, Jane M., "The Recognition of Psychosis in Non-Western Societies," in *Critical Issues in Psychiatric Diagnosis* (see ref. 3), pp. 1–13.
8. Chess, Stella, "Follow-up report on Autism in Congenital Rubella, *Journal of Autism and Childhood Schizophrenia* **7,** 69–81 (1977). See also: Stubbs, E. G., Ibid. **6,** 269–74.
9. McCusick, V. A., *Mendelian Inheritance in Man: Catalogues of Autosomal Dominant, Autosomal Recessive, and X-Linked Phenotypes,* 4th ed., Johns Hopkins University Press, Baltimore, 1975.
10. Friedberg, J., *Shock Treatment is Not Good for Your Brain,* Glide Publications, San Francisco, 1976.
11. "As Empty as Eve," *New Yorker,* 84–100 (9 Sept., 1974).
12. Davis, John M., "Overview: Maintenance Therapy in Psychiatry. II. Affective Disorders," *American Journal of Psychiatry* **133,** 1–13 (1976).
13. Mendels, J., "Lithium in the Treatment of Depression, Ibid., **133,** 373–378 (1976); also, F. Quitkin, et al., "On Prophylaxis in Unipolar Affective Disorder," Ibid. **133,** 250–260 (1976).
14. Jefferson, J. W., and Greist, J. H., *Primer of Lithium Therapy,* Williams and Wilkins, Baltimore, 1977. p. 33.

15. Hoffer, A., and Osmond, H., *How to Live with Schizophrenia,* Johnson, London, 1976.
16. Hawkins, D., and Pauling, L., *Orthomolecular Psychiatry,* Freeman, San Francisco, 1973.

Chapter 6

1. Glasser, see chapter 3, ref. 5.
2. Cooper, I. S., *The Victim is Always the Same,* Harper and Row, New York, 1973.
2a. Medawar, P. B., "Victims of Psychiatry." *New York Rev Books,* Jan. 23, 1975. Also, *The Hope of Progress,* Wildwood House, London, 1974.
4. Tennov, Dorothy, *Psychotherapy, the Hazardous Cure,* Abelard-Schuman, New York, 1975.
5. Hadley, Susan, W., and Strupp, Hans H., "Contemporary Views of Negative Effects in Psychotherapy," *Archives of General Psychiatry* **33,** 1291–1302 (1976).
6. Kahne, Merton J., "Suicide Among Patients in Mental Hospital: A Study of the Psychiatrists who Conducted their Psychotherapy," *Psychiatry* **31,** 32–42 (1968).
7. Light, Donald W., Jr., "Psychiatry and Suicide: The Management of a Mistake," *American Journal of Sociology* **77,** 821–839 (1972).
8. Henn, Ralph H., "Patient Suicide as Part of Psychiatric Residency," *Psychiatry* **135,** 745–746 (June, 1978).
9. Maugham, Somerset, *The Summing Up,* Penguin, New York, 1946, p. 7.
10. Freeman, John M., et al., "Folate-responsive homocystinuria and 'Schizophrenia'." *New England J. Med.* **292, 491–496 (1975).**

Chapter 7

1. Koranyi, E. K., "Morbidity and Rate of Undiagnosed Physical Illnesses in a Psychiatric Clinic Population," *Archives of General Psychiatry,* **36,** 414–419 (April, 1979).

2. Hall, R. C., et al., "Physical Illnesses Presenting as Psychiatric Diseases," Ibid. **35,** 1315–1320 (Nov., 1978).
3. Cerkez, C. T., and Ferguson, K. G., "Diabetes Mellitus with Secondary Hypoglycemia Simulating a Neuropsychiatric Disorder," C.M.A. *Journal* **92,** 1270–1273 (1965).
4. See ref. 9, chapter 4.
5. Fieve, R. R., "The Lithium Clinic: A New Model for the Delivery of Psychiatric Services, *The American Journal of Psychiatry* **132,** 1018–1022 (1975).

Chapter 8

1. Cowie, Valerie, *Genetics of Reading and Learning Difficulties,* a lecture delivered at the Health Sciences Center, University of British Columbia, May 20, 1976.
2. Hawkins, David R., "Impressions of Psychiatric Education in Western European Specialty Education," *Archives of General Psychiatry,* **36,** 713–717 (June, 1979).
3. Hirsch, S., "Observations on the Identity Problems of Psychiatrists," C.M.A. *Journal* **109,** 1090–1094 (1973).
4. See chapter 14, ref. 4, p. 749.
5. Spitzer, R. L., and Klein, D. F., *Evaluation of Psychological Therapies,* Johns Hopkins University Press, 1976, pp. 175–176.
6. Hippocrates, "On the Sacred Disease," in *Ancient Medicine and Other Treatises,* Francis Adams, translator, Regnery, 1949, p. 124.
7. Vincent, M. O., "Help Stamp out Psychiatrists," *Canadian Family Physician,* 69–71 (March, 1973).
8. Hackett, Thomas, "The Psychiatrist: In the Mainstream or on the Banks of Medicine?" *American Journal of Psychiatry* **134,** 432–434 (1977).
9. Rome, H. P., "Psychiatry and Foreign Affairs: The expanding competence of psychiatry, *American Journal of Psychiatry* **125,** 725–730 (1968).
10. See ref. 3.
11. See ref. 5, chapter 6.
12. May, Philip, R. A., *Treatment of Schizophrenia.* Science House, New York, 1968.

13. Marcus, A. M., et al., "The Psychologist as Primary Therapist—a Practical Consequence of the Concept of Health Sciences," *Canada's Mental Health* **26,** 12–14 (Sept., 1978).
14. Stone, Alan, *APA Newsletter,* Jan. 6, 1978.
15. Damunde, Earl, "The Militant Paraprofessionals: They Want a Slice of the Medicare Pie Now," *The Medical Post,* October 10, 1978, p. 13.
16. See ref. 3.
17. See ref. 3, chapter 6.
18. Gross, Martin L., *The Psychological Society,* Random House, New York and Toronto, 1978, p. 162.
19. Farrelly, Frank, and Brandsma, Jeff, *Provocative Therapy,* Shields, San Francisco, 1974.

Chapter 9

1. Adler, Alfred, *The Practice and Theory of Individual Psychology,* Kegan Paul, London, 1924, p. 35.
2. Freud, Sigmund, *New Introductory Lectures on Psychoanalysis,* Norton, New York, 1933, p. 181.
3. Ibid., p. 184.
4. Chesler, Phyllis, *Women and Madness,* Avon, New York, 1972.
5. See ref. 7, chapter 11.
6. See chapter 2, ref. 2, p. 170.
7. Floyd, William, "A New Look at Research in Marital and Family Therapy," *J. Family Counselling* **4,** 19–23 (1976).
8. See ref. 5, chapter 7.
9. *Diagnostic and Statistical Manual III,* American Psychiatric Association, in preparation.

Chapter 10

1. See chapter 16, footnote, p. 12.
2. See ref. 5, chapter 7.

3. Illych, Ivan, *Medical Nemesis,* Calder and Boyars, London, 1975.
4. Cooper, I. S., *The Victim is Always the Same,* Harper and Row, New York, 1973, p. xv.

Chapter 11

1. Kraepelin, E., "Patterns of Mental Disorder (translation), in *Themes and Variations in European Psychiatry,* Hirsch, S. R., and Shepherd, M., eds., Wright, Bristol, p. 7.
2. Gjessing, R., "Disturbances of Somatic Functions in Catatonia with a Periodic Course and their Compensation," *Journal of Mental Science* **84,** 608–619 (1938).
3. *White paper: Review of the Mental Health Act 1959,* Cmnd 7320, H. M. Stationery Office, London, 1978.
4. Meissner, W. W., "Thinking about the Family—Psychiatric Aspects," *Family Process* **3,** 1–40 (1964); see p. 3.
5. Ibid., pp. 16, 29.
6. Guerin, Philip J., Jr., ed., *Family Therapy: Theory and Practice,* Gardner Press, New York, 1976. p. 250.
7. Ibid., p. 27.
8. Time. July 5, 1968. Pg. 64–65
9. Kanner, L., *Nervous Child* **2,** 217 (1943).
10. Rimland, B., "Freud is Dead: New Dimensions in the Treatment of Mentally Ill Children, University of Southern California Distinguished Lecture Series in Special Education, June 1970. pp 33–48. See pg. 45.
11. Bettelheim, Bruno, *The Empty Fortress.* The Free Press, N. Y. 1967
12. (a) "Editorial," *British Medical Journal* **1972** (November 18), 379–80;
    (b) Cantwell, D. P., et al., "Families of Autistic and Dysphasic Children. I. Family Life and Interaction Patterns," *Archives of General Psychiatry* **36,** 682–687 (June, 1979).

13. See ref. 6, p. 250.
14. Pines, M., *Life* **71,** 67 (17 Dec., 1971).

Chapter 13

1. "When Thin Seems Fat," *Rassegna Medica* **LII,** 11–12 (1975).
2. Beiser, M., and Jilek-Aall, Group Leaders of the Workshop on the Healing Arts: East and West, described in *NIMH Newsletter,* March 1977, p. 2.
3. Hippocrates. See chapter 8, ref. 6, p. 123.

Chapter 14

1. Meyler, L., *Side Effects of Drugs,* Excerpta Medica Foundation, Amsterdam, 1975.
2. Wechsler, James, *In a Darkness,* Norton, 1972.
3. Wilson, Louise, G. P. Putnam, 1968.
4. Quitkin, F., Rifkin, A., and Klein, D. F., "Monoamine Oxidase Inhibitors: A Review of Antidepressant Effectiveness," *Archives of General Psychiatry* **36,** 749–760 (1979).
5. Kraft, D. P., and Haroutun, M. B., "Suicide by Persons with and without Psychiatric Contacts," *Archives of General Psychiatry* **33,** 209–215 (1976).
6. Myers, D. H., and Neal, C. D., "Suicide in Psychiatric Patients," *British Journal of Psychiatry* **133,** 38–44 (1978).
7. Copas, J. B., et al., "Danger Periods for Suicide in Patients Under Treatment," *Psychological Medicine* **1,** 400–404 (1971). Synopsis: "Using statistical methods, the hypothesis that suicide occurs either at the beginning or at the end of a spell of treatment is shown to fit the available data."
8. Barraclough, B., et al., "A Hundred Cases of Suicide: Clinical Aspects," *British Journal of Psychiatry* **125,** 355–373 (1974).
9. See ref. 4.

Chapter 15

1. See chapter 8, ref. 5, Preface.
2. See chapter 6, ref. 5.
3. *Encounter Groups and Psychiatry.* Task Force Report of the American Psychiatric Association, Irving D. Yalom, Chairman, American Psychiatric Association, Washington, 1970.
4. McCord, Joan, "Thirty-year Followup: Counselling Fails," *Science News* **112,** 357 (1977).
5. Sullivan, H. S., *The Interpersonal Theory of Psychiatry,* Norton, New York, 1953, p. 309.
6. Milgram, Stanley, *Obedience to Authority: an Experimental View,* Harper and Row, New York, 1974.
7. Berenson, B. G., "Confrontation: Those Who Qualify and Those who Don't," *Canadian Counsellor* **8,** 121–125 (1974).
8. Schutz, W., *Joy: Expanding Human Awareness,* Grove, New York, 1967.
9. Mintz, Alan L., "Encounter Groups and Other Panaceas," *Commentary* 42–49 (1973).
10. See ref. 7.
11. Kaplan, H. S., Sadock, "Structured Interaction: A New Technique in Group Psychotherapy," *American Journal of Psychotherapy* **25,** 418–427 (1971).
12. See ref. 6, Chapter 3.
13. Karasu, Toksoz B., "Psychotherapies: an Overview," *American Journal of Psychiatry* **134,** 851–863 (1977).
14. See chapter 3, ref. 2, p. 322.
15. See chapter 6, ref. 2.
16. "Live and Let Live," *New Yorker,* 82–87, (July 16, 1979).
17. Gross, Martin, L., *The Psychological Society,* Random House, New York. 1978, p. 140.
18. Martin, D. C., et al., "Human Subjects in Clinical Research—A Report of Three Studies," *New England J. Med.* **279,** 1426–1431 (1968).
19. Brackbill, Yvonne, and Golden, Lori, "Public Opinion on Subject Participation in Biomedical Research: New Views on Altruism, Perception of Risk, and Proxy Consent," *Clinical Res.* **27,** 14–18 (Feb. 1979).

Chapter 16

1. Miller, Henry, "The Abuse of Psychiatry," *Encounter,* **34,** 24–31 (May, 1970); see p. 24.
2. Ibid., p. 28.
3. Murray, Robin M., "A Reappraisal of American Psychiatry," *Lancet,* i, 255–258, (3 February, 1979).